The Logic Diet

The Logic Diet

♦

How Very Large People Can Lose
50 To 100 Pounds Or More And
Keep It Off Forever
(It Can Work For Smaller People Too!)

Russell J. Lawrence

iUniverse, Inc.
New York Lincoln Shanghai

The Logic Diet
How Very Large People Can Lose 50 To 100 Pounds Or More And Keep It Off Forever (It Can Work For Smaller People Too!)

Copyright © 2006 by Russell J. Lawrence

All rights reserved. No part of this book may be used or reproduced by any means, graphic, electronic, or mechanical, including photocopying, recording, taping or by any information storage retrieval system without the written permission of the publisher except in the case of brief quotations embodied in critical articles and reviews.

iUniverse books may be ordered through booksellers or by contacting:

iUniverse
2021 Pine Lake Road, Suite 100
Lincoln, NE 68512
www.iuniverse.com
1-800-Authors (1-800-288-4677)

You should not undertake any diet/exercise regimen recommended in this book before consulting your personal physician. Neither the author nor the publisher shall be responsible or liable for any loss or damage allegedly arising as a consequence of your use or application of any information or suggestions contained in this book.

ISBN-13: 978-0-595-41884-8 (pbk)
ISBN-13: 978-0-595-86232-0 (ebk)
ISBN-10: 0-595-41884-8 (pbk)
ISBN-10: 0-595-86232-2 (ebk)

Printed in the United States of America

To my wife Milissa and my sons Parker and Evan, all the inspiration I need.

Contents

Foreword...ix
Introduction..xi
Set Your Goal...1
Stage 1: Cut Out The Fat..3
- *The Logic Behind Stage 1*.......................................5
- *Supplements*..7
- *You Will Have To Give Up Foods You Love*.......................9
- *Cooking for Yourself Is Not Hard!*.............................11
- *My Favorite Fat Free Foods*....................................13
- *Cheating On Stage 1*...27
- *Does Stage 1 Have To End?*.....................................28

Stage 2: No More Eating Late.....................................30
- *What is Late?*...31
- *The Logic Behind Stage 2*......................................32
- *Tricks Of The Trade*...33
- *Eat Dinner Right Before Your Time Deadline*...................34
- *Acceptable Snacks If You're Going To Crack*...................36
- *Cheating on Stage 2*...38
- *The Math Of Cheating*..40
- *When Does Stage 2 End?*..41

Stage 3: Reduce Portions...42
- *The Logic Behind Stage 3*......................................44
- *Quantifying Stage 3*...46

- *Cheating On Stage 3*...... 47
- *When Does Stage 3 End (And Does It Have To)?*...... 49
- *Gearing Up For Stage 4*...... 51

Stage 4: Counting Calories (The Right Way)...... 52
- *The Results Are In The Math*...... 54
- *The Exercise Factor*...... 56
- *The Logic Behind Stage 4*...... 58
- *The Importance Of Serving Size*...... 60
- *Don't Leave Anything Out*...... 62
- *Planning The Day*...... 63
- *Cheating On Stage 4*...... 67
- *The End Of Stage 4 (A Monumental Occasion!)*...... 69
- *Another Look At Plateaus*...... 72
- *Review Before Moving Forward*...... 75

Stage 5: Maintaining Your New Body...... 77
- *A New Goal Means New Math*...... 78
- *The Logic Behind Stage 5*...... 79
- *Moderation Takes Baby Steps*...... 81
- *The Last Of The Baby Steps*...... 85
- *Cheating On Stage 5*...... 87
- *Final Weight-Loss Words*...... 89

Stage 6: Spicing Things Back Up...... 91
- *There Can Be Variety In Healthy Eating*...... 92
- *You're A Cook Now…Right?!*...... 93
- *Cheating On Stage 6*...... 95
- *Remember To Spot Check*...... 96

Conclusion...... 99

Before And After Photos...... 101

Foreword

I'm a big guy. I currently stand 6'2" and weigh in at 186 lbs. I *used* to be a big **<u>FAT</u>** guy, weighing in at a whopping 268 lbs.! That's right, I lost 82 pounds, and as of this moment, I've kept it off for over a year and a half (and counting!).

I didn't do *Weight Watchers*. I didn't do *Adkins*. I didn't do *Jenny Craig* or *Trimspa*. In fact, I didn't do ***any*** prescribed diet plan whatsoever. What I did was to make up my own plan and adapt it as I went along. This plan was based totally on my logical idea of what should work for a guy my size in order to get me where I wanted to be for the rest of my life, while not driving me crazy with hunger in the process.

It sounds easy to say that you need to eat right, exercise, cut calories, and basically change everything you're used to doing. We all know it's **<u>NOT</u>** easy. Of course, we've all tried to do it many times, and we may have had some short successes. However, we've always gained the weight back, and sometimes become even heavier than before we started.

I need to specify now that I am not a doctor. I am not a fitness trainer. I am not trained in any art or science pertaining to the body or weight control. I'm just a regular guy who got big and fat by not eating the proper foods and eating way too much of the other foods.

I didn't care at what time of day I ate or if I skipped breakfast. I didn't exercise. Heck, I was even smoking 2 packs of cigarettes a day back then as well (I quit in September of 2003, but that's another story). All it took was for me to make up my mind that I really ***wanted*** to lose the weight and get healthier. That's when I started my plan.

The Stages of my plan are set up to ***easily*** and ***gradually*** guide people who are significantly overweight or obese into changing their daily habits, changing the foods they eat, changing how much they eat, and changing when they eat. I promise that if my methods are followed, not only will you lose the weight and set yourself up to keep it off forever, but you'll be ***absolutely delighted*** as you see how you can keep full and enjoy much more flexibility than other diets along your journey.

This is not to say that my diet plan would not work for women, smaller people, or people who want to lose 10 to 30 vanity pounds. ***IT WILL WORK FOR***

YOU TOO! All you have to do is skip to the last few stages of my plan instead of starting at the beginning.

If you only have 10 or 20 pounds to lose, you most likely are already exercising or using a healthier menu and don't need to be gradually led to my final stages, which require more control than most excessively large people have.

My plan takes advantage of the fact that, in this day and age, the amount of products manufactured for the consumer that are low in fat or completely fat free are unbelievably HUGE compared to even a few years ago, and are getting more plentiful and better tasting every day. The availability of these foods makes the task of converting to healthier foods much less stressful.

I will show you how to use these products to help you change your life forever. With the proper plan in place, using the proper tools and methods, you are guaranteed success.

Lastly I will say that I challenge any doctor or diet review network to read my plan and assess its health value for the user. Exercise, though recommended, is ***not required*** in order to achieve amazing results with my plan. Even so, I firmly believe that my diet is one of the healthier plans out there, both for the mind and body, and that, when reviewed, will generate glowing remarks.

I'm not a psychologist either, but conditioning the mind into converting from thinking like an overweight person into thinking like a thin person, without driving you crazy in the process, is of the utmost importance for a weight-loss program to be permanently successful. Most plans leave this important factor out of the mix!

Many of the principles I've used are not new, they're tried and true pieces of the healthy lifestyle puzzle. What *is* new is how I've put that puzzle together in a way to make it much easier for anyone to get the desired results from those pieces.

Try my plan and you'll become a fan. I promise!

Russell J. Lawrence

Introduction

I'm writing this introduction to my diet plan so you can read about my motivations to start doing it and to give you my story so you can see that, if I can do this, anyone can do this!

I have always been overweight...not to the extent I was when I started this plan, but I had fought the big gut for many years. I used the *Slim Fast* diet plan to lose 50 pounds back in my college days, only to gain it back once I started eating real food again.

You see, I was one of those people who ate like a professional football player at every meal, every day. I used to win money in eating contests at school (going back to the eighth grade!). I never ate a real breakfast. Sometimes, I would eat several doughnuts or pastries if they were presented to me at a class or work function. Other times, I would eat cookies or even candy bars to start off my day.

My idea of a regular lunch was 2 or 3 double cheeseburgers, a large fries, and a super-size Pepsi. Maybe I would go to an all-you-can-eat place for lunch. Hometown Buffet or any Chinese buffets were normal stops. If I were on a dare, I'd eat 2 or even 3 Wendy's ***triples*** and even finish off the Biggie fries and drink.

Dinner would always come late, say between 7 and 9 PM, and would be whatever I could find, usually frozen pizzas, or maybe even more fast food. I might just make a pile of nachos and sit in front of the TV and watch a baseball game while stuffing my face. By 10:30 or 11:00 PM, I'd be eating dessert, probably more cookies, brownies, ice cream, or maybe a different kind of chips. I loved to eat cheese cubes or just melt them on toast for a quick grilled cheese sandwich. Peanut butter on Nilla Wafers was also a favorite. Then I'd go to bed, wake up the next morning, and start all over again.

You see, most people out there can't relate to what I'm talking about. They think you can just cut back or count calories and start losing weight. That's because they don't eat the sheer quantities of bad foods that some of us big people eat. I'm not saying that everyone eats like I used to, but for those of you out there that do, or those that are close, you can understand what I was like. Some of you know what I mean when I describe eating whatever you want, whenever you want. You eat junk and candy all day long at work, then fast food and pizza at night.

If you do cook your own dinners, it's a load of pasta and garlic bread or anything with a ton of melted cheese all over it. You always have to have that full feeling at every meal, so you stuff yourself.

When I met my wife I was 24 years old and overweight with a smoking habit. She loved me for who I was and what I looked like. As the years went by I got bigger and fatter, my pants size went up and up in the waist, yet my wife continued to stay attracted to me. I was, and am, extremely lucky to have such a woman at my side.

Now, I **knew** I was overweight and unhealthy. I **told myself** that **someday** I'd get back to a slimmer build and healthier lifestyle. In reality, I just didn't care, and could always find a rationalization for continuing on the path I was traveling. I believe that all of you reading this **know** you have a problem and truly **want** to fix it. I just believe you think you'll fail, and have failed before, so just don't try that hard anymore.

That's exactly how I was.

In July of 2001, my wife became pregnant with our fist son, who we named Parker. I thought about what would happen when he turned 3 years old and wanted to start playing baseball or even just running around the backyard kicking a soccer ball. I realized that, at the pace I was going, I would not be able to do all of those things with him, and much worse, might not even be around for him in the long term, since I was basically a heart attack waiting to happen.

I put together my 5-year plan to stop smoking, lose weight, and get into better shape. I'll not go into my smoking cessation plan, but it worked. By October 2003, I had quit smoking. My son was going on 18 months old at that time. By February 2004, I was ready to start the diet I had planned for almost 3 years.

Whatever your motivation for being at this step, I applaud you. It takes guts to decide to better yourself, no matter what the reason. I'm glad that I can make this easier for you, and that I did all the planning for you, so you won't have to wait a few years to get going. Let my work be your guide, and your success is foolproof. I'll even give you the tips for cheating on my diet so you can have fun once in awhile!

Good luck to you! Let's begin.

Set Your Goal

OK, you're 50 to 100 pounds overweight (or more). You're a big person and you know it. You eat a *LOT* of food and you know it. You **MUST** set a goal for yourself right now, before you get started. My initial goal was to get to 215 lbs. That would have been a 53-pound loss, and I thought it'd be very hard to get there. So I'm glad I ended up changing that to 205, then 195, and then finally 190!

If you used to be thinner, set the goal for when you were 15 pounds above your thinnest. Whatever you decide, know that the goal can be changed lower in the future, but *not* higher! Make the goal low enough to be very challenging in your mind. You'll be even more gratified when you reach it.

Understand that this is going to take some time. There is no pressure on my plan, at least in Stages 1–3, to get to a certain level by a certain date. Do not make the mistake of stressing yourself based on time. If you are starting at Stage 1 of my plan, you need to lose a lot more than vanity pounds, and must make much bigger strides in changing your entire lifestyle to get the job done.

This is going to take time! You can't say "I need to be in Speedos by the end of the summer," or anything like that! If you're looking to shed a few vanity pounds, go directly to Stage 4 of my plan.

A secondary goal you should set for yourself is to get through Stage 1 without cheating once. After Stage 1, I will get into the cheating allowances as it starts to get a little more difficult, but Stage 1 is so easy, and you get to stay full, so you shouldn't deviate from the path at all.

Once you've got these goals engrained in your brain, it's time to set a start date. I don't think you should start as soon as you read this chapter. I believe you should prepare yourself, if even for a day or two, before rolling with the new diet.

When I quit smoking, I had the exact date planned in advance for months. The night before, I smoked several packs as a "last hurrah" so to speak. I did the same thing with the diet. I started on an exact day, and ate my face off the day before. I went out with no regrets!

Notice here that I'm not asking you to set a goal for exercise. You will continue to see that theme throughout this book. No exercise is necessary for my plan to work. I repeat…**NO EXERCISE IS NECESSARY FOR MY PLAN TO WORK.**

I am **NOT** saying you shouldn't exercise! I started exercising regularly by the end of Stage 3. I did not use a gym or anything like that. I bought a bike and started taking nightly bike rides with my son in the child seat. Then I bought a basketball hoop for my driveway and, to this day, try to get in 20–45 minutes every night of basketball. That is the extent of my exercise. Hopefully, any doctor would tell you that these forms of exercise are as good as any other and great for long-term health if done consistently.

Working out with weights does build more muscle, which does help you burn fat and raise your metabolism, but I'm not going to tell you to do it! Forget about the exercise for now, unless you really want to of course. The more you do, the faster you will see the results, but here in the cold, Midwest winters, I did nothing at all during those months, and still lost the weight almost as fast.

Lastly, you should set the expectation that you may, or may not, get help and assistance from your family, friends and co-workers. Understand that your spouse or significant other, your kids if you have them, your friends, and the people around you every day, are *not* usually going to change themselves **one iota** in response to what you're doing.

If you have loving people that will keep temptation away from you in order to help you, then you are truly a blessed individual. Otherwise, expect those around you to continue eating junk food in front of you, having late night snacks around you, and even asking you to join them, seemingly with malice toward your attempt at bettering yourself!

You must understand that you are making a significant change and those around you don't have (or need) the willpower to do so as well. You *MUST* take pride in what you are doing and know that, once you've started to show results, these people will become jealous of you. Many will come to admire you. Others will tell you that it'll never last, and then be put in their place a year later.

Also remember that the opposite sex will look at you a lot differently as well (and that's in a positive way!), so keep focused. My plan will make this easier for you than any other, so you can feel well prepared, and I'll give you many ways to combat those temptations.

So if you're ready, it's time to get started.

Stage 1

Cut Out The Fat

OK, so how do we get started? It's as simple as the chapter title says…cut out the fat. That's right, I mean zero fat grams every day (or as close as you can get to it). If impossible to do zero, then the absolute maximum to be allowed is 25 grams.

I'll next say that you can eat *anything* you want, *as much* as you want, *at any time* you want, as long as you follow the fat gram rule.

Sound simple? It is! Sound tough to you? It's **NOT!** Everything you can buy has nutritional labels. The only items that usually don't are fruits and vegetables, which are fat free, so for now, you can eat all the fruits and vegetables you want!

The only reason I'm allowing up to 25 grams of fat is to allow meat at dinnertime that isn't fat free bologna (yes they make fat free bologna!) so you can get a good amount of protein. A regular size boneless, skinless chicken breast has only about 6 grams of fat, while providing about 36 grams of protein. I'm not saying this is a protein diet! I'm just saying I'll give you a little bit of fat if you want to get some extra protein!

Now, you're thinking this might be no bargain. Maybe you think it's no big deal to be able to eat all the low or non-fat stuff you want because you think you won't find anything good. Well think again.

I'm going to tell you some of the things you can shoot for in this Stage, but honestly, it'll be more fun for you to find out for yourself. Go through every aisle of the supermarket and look for fat free items. Try any that look interesting. Every meal is represented by fat free stuff at the store, including yummy snacks. I guarantee it!

I will be honest now and say that this is not going to be cheap. Generally speaking, the lower fat and fat free products you find at the market will be more expensive than their fattening, sugar-filled counterparts. I look at it this way…the amount of money you're saving by not ordering fast food and pizza all the time, as well as all the junk food and candy you're not buying, will be replaced by the amount you'll spend on eating the low fat foods. It will seem very expensive, but just remember what you're ***not*** buying anymore.

Also, many people are spending money on home gyms, exercise equipment, personal trainers, expensive diet pills, herbal remedies, and the like. You are simply spending the money on more expensive food items, and the best part is that you get to eat them!

Of course, you aren't going to like everything you pick up at the store. I guarantee you, however, that you will end up ***loving*** many of them, and will end up buying them probably for the rest of your life!

Unfortunately many of the things you need to round out your meals might not be available at your local stores. In this case, I will tell you to go online to the company's website and have the stuff shipped to your door! I have done this in several cases with foods that were discontinued at my local supermarket. It actually helped me because I could order a larger quantity and have a supply in storage at the house.

I will tell you some of my favorites in a bit, but for now, try to become your own expert. Try to find out as many foods as you can on your own. Make it fun! Make a game out of it for your family the next time you're at the store!

THE LOGIC BEHIND STAGE 1

OK, you're saying, "why is this going to work?" So since this is based on my logic, I'll tell you how I thought it through.

Stage 1 is, again, designed for very large people at least 50 to 100 pounds overweight like I was when I started. People like that eat large quantities of all the wrong foods and love every minute of it. When you break this down even a little, you'd estimate that most of you are eating probably 6,000 to 20,000 calories a day! Some of you maybe even *more* than that! Also, the amounts of fat grams in your daily diet are probably so many, that it'd be horrifying to even know the truth.

Therefore, if you eat the same large quantity of food, but make sure that none of it is high in fat, you'll guarantee yourself that you're also eating a lot fewer calories and grams of sugar as well, since the lower fat foods are also mostly lower in those areas.

You're basically just living the lesser of two evils at first, and since the first evil was *so* bad for you, the lesser evil ends up reaping a vast improvement in your weight, and also your health! You *are* eating healthier foods (at least healthier than the ones you *were* eating), just a lot of them. Since a lot of the better foods will affect you so much less than a lot of the bad foods, you lose weight. It's that simple!

Believe me, the skinnier people will be very jealous of you. You will be able to tell everyone how you've lost 25 pounds, and you still eat all day and all night! This is simply because you were so large and ate so much before, that it's easy to drop a bunch of pounds with this little effort at first.

What you're also doing with Stage 1 however, is setting yourself up mentally for what is to come. You're letting yourself down gradually in order to get to the next level, and can still eat a lot, and keep yourself feeling full, while doing it!

Oh, and by now, you'll notice I haven't mentioned one word about carbs or limiting them in any way. That's because I don't care about carbs and neither should you! Eat all the carbs you want as long as they're a part of those non-fat or low-fat foods. They simply do not hinder your ability to lose weight. In fact, I believe they help you to feel full, and help keep your cravings for all those other foods to a much lower level while you're adjusting to the new lifestyle.

What makes you lose weight is simply the reduction in calories you're eating in relation to the calories you're burning. **<u>PERIOD!</u>**

You'll notice once you start keeping track of nutritional information in Stage 4, that as you keep eating better and better foods, the carbs will naturally start to come down as well (along with many other bad influences on your body).

SUPPLEMENTS

At this point, I'm going to discuss the supplements I take and the logic behind me taking them every day. I do not take any strange herbal remedies or fad pills to help me lose weight. You should not need any expensive weight loss aids or the like on my plan. You can eat a lot of food so you won't need appetite suppressants.

Even before I was doing my diet, I was taking 1000 mg of Vitamin C each morning. I was doing this with the hope that it would help me not get sick as much. You see, I was always catching every bug out there and had the flu twice per year, etc. I couldn't tell you if it really works, but I don't feel it could hurt and I still take this every morning to this day.

I will say that I did not start taking any other supplements until Stage 4 of my plan, but if I had read up on them sooner, I would have started at Stage 1, so you can benefit from this now.

After reading many articles in many magazines such as *Men's Health*, *Woman's World*, and others, I began taking a daily multivitamin. With everything written out there to back it up, I think this is a no-brainer and you should start immediately. The one I chose, and still use every day, is One-A-Day Weight Smart, but you can choose whichever you like.

For a while, I was taking a cinnamon tablet supplement, about 500 mg per day. I read somewhere that it would help keep my blood sugar levels in balance while I cut so much sugar from my diet. I don't know if it really did anything and I stopped taking them in Stage 5, but you may read up on this and find it might help you.

Lastly, I take 1000 mg of Calcium fortified with 400 IU of Vitamin D for absorption every day and I firmly believe you should too. Some might say it's too much and that a lot will just pass through your system, but I started doing this in Stage 4 and I personally saw the weight just start pouring off my body.

The interesting thing to me is that I read somewhere, I think in *Woman's World*, that the next big diet craze that will hit this country in the future will consist of mostly dairy, and that high calcium will be seen as a huge factor in helping to lose weight. This is the same thinking on taking 3 servings of fat free yogurt each day. I'm a believer!

That's it! I take nothing else! However, I will say that I religiously take these pills each morning, every morning, without fail. Whether or not I am taking the day off my plan for a cheat day, I will take the supplements. I do **REQUIRE** that you take at least the multivitamin and calcium starting in Stage 4, and I *strongly* *suggest* you start right now in order to get used to it and get the habit down cold. You can't skip or forget. I promise you'll see quicker weight loss results when you're taking them as well. I can't back that up with science, but I watched it work!

As a last thought here, I have not had a cold, the flu, or any virus at all affect me, no matter how many people around me were sick with it, since November, 2004 (I started my diet in February, 2004!). That's almost 2 years without being sick. Coincidence?

Alright, after all of this, the following statement should have been in the back of your mind this whole time, and now it needs to be brought to the forefront:

You Will Have To Give Up Foods You Love

I will show you that there are many wonderful foods you can eat that are low in fat or fat free, but there are simply some things that our scientists have not yet figured out how to make low fat for us, so I'm going to break your hearts a little bit here and list some of the things that you absolutely ***must not eat.***

- All fast food (there are a slight few exceptions, but not worth exploring until stage 5 or 6, so for now, absolutely all must be avoided)

- All Pizza

- Regular cheese (any kind)

- Regular milk

- All regular soda pop (no fat, but will KILL you on sugar and calories later, so give it up NOW!)

- Regular bread (all kinds, including bagels, etc.)

- All hard candy (like pop, it's fat free, but you can't get used to eating it so stop NOW!)

- All soft candy and candy bars

- All chocolate

- All doughnuts and pastries

- All regular muffins, cakes, etc.

- All regular burgers and hot dogs

- All ribs, bacon, sausage, pork products (unless *extremely* lean pork chops)

- All peanut butter

- All regular jams and jellies

- All regular mayonnaise and other fattening condiments

- Regular salad dressings

- All regular syrups (any kind whether chocolate or maple!)

- Regular butter and margarines

I could make this list go on and on and probably fill many pages of all the stuff you *can't* eat. I just wanted to list the major items here and make sure you understand that all of these things are the main reason you got really heavy in the first place. You eat a lot of fattening foods, and then top them off with all kinds of ***extremely*** fattening condiments too!

Now you'll also notice that I keep using the word *"regular"* in the list above. This should give you hope for what comes next! Many of those foods and condiments you crave are out there in the stores right now waiting for you in fat free versions! Some things there are no hope for like pizza and peanut butter. You have to realize that you (if you are ***truly*** serious about this) will ***never*** be eating these things on a regular basis again.

Now before you start yelling…I know and you know that the fat free versions of a lot of things have a stigma to them. People don't think they taste as good and think that some taste just downright awful. Well no matter what you've heard or what you think, I'm here to tell you the following:

1) **OF COURSE** these things aren't going to taste the same or as good as the bad stuff. If they did, there would be no bad stuff out there and we'd all be eating fat free, vitamin-fortified double cheeseburgers at McDonalds.

2) The technology and abilities of those out there that are manufacturing these products has gotten ***much*** better over the last 5 years. These foods and condiments taste amazingly good compared to what they used to taste like, and they're getting better tasting every day. There are also more and more choices seemingly every week at the market due to the tendency in this country toward better health and the population trying to buck the obesity trend.

3) Last and most important. ***JUST DEAL WITH IT!*** If you don't want to be ***fat*** anymore, you will have to learn to love these foods, be excited about shopping for these foods, and create tasty combinations of these foods that you'll look forward to eating for the rest of your life if necessary. I can personally attest to the fact that I now have favorites I've been eating for 2 years or more and I'm not going to stop because I love them so much. I look forward to eating these foods every day, and I swear you will as well if you give them the chance!

COOKING FOR YOURSELF IS NOT HARD!

Another thing you're going to have to deal with now is that you'll have to start cooking your own meals. Healthy, thinner people are not going out to eat very often at all and are certainly not eating pre-packaged foods very often either. No more TV dinners!

There are a few diet plans out there including *Jenny Craig* and *Nutrisystem* that take advantage of you out there who are unwilling, or *think* are unable, to cook your own meals. These plans are very expensive and make it impossible for you, in my opinion, to keep the weight off once you lose it. What are you expected to do, eat the food they send you every day for the rest of your life? You need to learn to cook for yourself anyway once it's all over!

Look, I am a guy. My wife does not cook. In fact, she works nights and I work days, so I have to do this for myself no matter what I want. I am not predisposed to cooking. I would much prefer not to have to do it. I'm not going to tell you I use a bunch of pre-preparation methods to have stuff ready all week, because I don't. What I will tell you is that you do not need to be a master of the oven or have read up on culinary mastery techniques.

If I can learn to prepare my own meals then anyone can do it. I'm going to make this really simple for you like the rest of my plan. For a big, overweight person like you, you're only going to need 4 or 5 cooking appliances in your arsenal in order to live very comfortably on this plan.

1) The oven. You will use this mostly for cooking and broiling fish. If you don't eat any fish, I'll bet you won't even need this appliance for a while!

2) The toaster. You'll be using this every morning for sure. I'm sure you can handle it.

3) The microwave. This is going to be your major staple of cooking every single day. You'll see in my future recipes and food listings that a lot of what you'll be doing will be in the microwave.

4) The stovetop. Throughout Stages 1, 2, and 3, you'll be using the stovetop a lot for making pasta and maybe corn and stuff like that. This isn't too tough either.

5) The number 1 appliance you'll need to get used to is an indoor grill. It doesn't have to be made by that big ex-boxer guy. It can be of any make or model. Once you learn to use this amazing piece of technology, you'll wonder how you ever lived without it. You can take lean burger patties and chicken breasts right out of the freezer, plop them directly on the grill, and let them cook

until done (usually 5–12 minutes depending on size and whether they're frozen or thawed before cooking).

Does this list and what's explained within it look daunting to you? I should hope not. Some of you big people out there probably got as big as you are because you've *never* been afraid to cook for yourself so this shouldn't be a problem.

For the rest of you, I assure you that once you start changing the foods you eat as part of this plan and begin to see the results, you're not going to mind having to prepare things. You'll see how easy it really is. I'll say again that thin people do this every day. You are changing your lifestyle and mentality overall over the life of this plan, so this is another small step that will get you there.

Also, spending more money on healthy foods will reassure you that you don't want to be spending any more money eating out or buying the more expensive pre-packaged foods anyway. You can't watch your fat grams while eating out at restaurants. You need to be in a controlled environment (your home!) in order to control what you eat.

MY FAVORITE FAT FREE FOODS

OK, if you want some help, here it comes. I'm not going to list the natural low fat and fat free foods here, you should know those (like fruits and vegetables, etc.) without me having to say. Also, if you're unsure about the fat content of natural foods or foods in the market which have no labels on them, you can go on the internet, do a web search on your favorite search engine for "calorie counters" or anything like that and find many free web pages that will allow you to look up any food out there (like a tomato for example) and get a nutritional label for it. My favorite is www.nutritiondata.com.

You will find this extremely handy later when you get to Stage 4, but for now, if you have any doubt as to the fat grams in something, go online!

Now, I'm going to be listing a lot of exact brand names here since these are many of the ones I've found, that I've taste tested, and that I love! This doesn't, of course, mean that *you'll* love them at all, and it also doesn't mean that you'll even be able to find them in your area of the country. If there are websites I've used to order them, I'll list them for you.

There may be other websites I don't even know about, so you can just search for them yourself! It's easy to order online and you get the right stuff delivered right to your door! There will also be some generic listings and you can select from the brands at your market.

I'm going to separate these into meal groups to make it easier for me. All of these you can use in Stage 1 through Stage 3! You can substitute different brands as long as they're fat free.

BREAKFAST

- Fat free Cool Whip
- Sugar Free Cool Whip
- Dannon Light 'N Fit Yogurt (any flavor!)
- Schwebel's Lite Wheat enriched bread (for toast)
- Parkay fat free butter spray
- Any fat free coffee creamer
- NatraTaste Zero Calorie Sweetener (less expensive than most others)

- Smuckers Sugar Free Jelly (any flavor)

- Sugar Free Jello cups

- Any fat free pudding cups (any flavor)

- Better 'n Eggs Healthier Real Egg Product (or any fat free egg substitute)

- Any fat free sliced cheese product (I like the sharp cheddar flavor made by my market, but Kraft has one as well)

- Any fat free crackers (any type) (low fat are OK, but be careful, the fat grams could add up quick and you need to stay under 25 per day, so I'd stick with the fat free)

- Any fat free milk

- Any fat free breakfast cereal! (there are SO many to choose from!)

- Any fat free sour cream

- Any fat free cream cheese spread

- Any sugar free, fat free angel food cake

- Any fat free cookies or muffins you can find

Again, this has not been even close to an all-inclusive list! You will find many other breakfast foods out there. I will now give some examples of what I would eat for breakfast.

By the way, you probably haven't been used to eating breakfast at all and maybe are saying to yourself that you're not going to start now since you're not hungry in the morning.

I'm here to tell you, *YOU'D BETTER START EATING BREAKFAST RIGHT NOW*, and I mean **EVERY SINGLE DAY.** It is crucial to this diet plan and most reading you can do out there about healthy lifestyles will tell you the same. Believe me, as you start to lose weight even in Stage 1 of my plan, you're going to be very grateful that you can eat a lot of food right when you get up in the morning and before you go to work.

You're not going to be eating a bunch of junk all day anymore to keep yourself full and you're not going to be having those big fattening lunches anymore either.

If you think your schedule doesn't allow for it, then get your butt up 15–30 minutes earlier than you normally do and *make time* for it. This is **REQUIRED.**

Here are just a couple of my breakfasts that I eat right now, and some I ate when I first started. Now this should still seem like a lot of food compared to what you were probably expecting, but remember, in Stage 1, if it's still not enough, you can make the quantities of these things as much as your mind, stomach, and wallet can deal with!

1) Coffee with fat free creamer and sugar substitute. Frozen mixed berries thawed in the microwave, drained, and placed in a bowl full of fat free Cool Whip then covered with a cup of fat free strawberry yogurt (this is unbelievable!). 2 slices of fat free toast with fat free butter spray and sugar free jelly.

2) Coffee (as above). Make ¼ cup of egg substitute as per directions, then put on toast with the butter spray and a slice of fat free cheese (only takes a few minutes and is awesome!). Make 2 of these sandwiches if you're hungry! 1 cup of fat free yogurt. Fresh strawberries dipped in fat free chocolate sauce (yes it's out there! You can use Hershey's syrup if you want!).

3) Coffee. Fat free crackers and fat free cheese. Berries (as above). Fat free pudding cups with fat free Cool Whip.

4) Coffee. Bowl of fat free cereal in fat free milk (or two…three?!). Cup of yogurt. Toast (as above).

5) Coffee. Bananas (1–2). Fat free cream cheese on fat free bagels (if you can find them) or fat free bread slices. Berries.

6) Coffee. Grapes. Toast (as above). Egg substitute (scrambled). Cup of yogurt.

7) Coffee. Fat free cookies or muffins. Berries. Banana.

8) Coffee. Fat free angel food cake. Berries.

As you can see, there are many variations and I could go on forever. You can make any combination of breakfast foods as you see fit and may find many other things I've not listed here.

You can also see I like coffee every morning but you can obviously substitute water, milk, or even diet pop if you wish. I would stay away from juices unless they're sugar free. You'll have to give them up later since they have a lot of calories anyway so don't get hooked on them.

One thing I will not deviate from is that you should most definitely have a cup of the yogurt every morning without fail. Whether it's by itself eaten with a spoon, or poured over my berries and Cool Whip concoction, you must do it. Along with the supplements I've suggested, remember that there's a lot of talk out there that yogurt and calcium are both great for helping you lose weight and burn fat at the same time. With the results I've seen, I'm not going to argue.

LUNCH

Are you one of those people who say "I don't eat lunch either," or "lunch is for wimps," or "I don't have time for lunch?" Well, I'm here to tell you that has to change also! Many diets and articles on the subject will tell you that eating many small meals throughout the day is better for you than 3 big meals. Now I'm not going to tell you to eat 6 times per day, because that won't work too well with my diet (you can do it if you want, but it'll make Stage 4 more taxing). However, just as you MUST eat breakfast, you **MUST EAT LUNCH ALSO.**

I'm not talking about going out to lunch either, or ordering in to your place of work. You are going to have to learn to, dare I say it, **pack** your lunch from home, bring it to where you work, put it in a refrigerator (or pack it in one of those lunch containers you can put ice packs in if you have no fridge access), and take it out during lunch time and eat it! Those of you who don't have to work during the day (or at all), this will be easy for you!

Don't want to do this? Then you've pretty much failed already. I know that sounds mean, but you simply must keep your metabolism charged during the day with good, healthy, low-fat foods. You did the right thing by charging up your metabolism at breakfast, so you've got to keep it going!

On the flip side, you simply **cannot** find any healthy food out there to order every day. Besides, you've already spent the extra money on good foods for the house, so instead of trying to spend more at lunchtime, pack the good stuff.

Think you don't have time to make lunch? Well, that extra time in the morning you've made to prepare and eat breakfast includes more than enough time to make and pack the lunch. I guarantee it!

Here is the list of the lunch items I use now and have used in the early Stages if you want to join me. Remember, this is not all-inclusive and you can find all of your own at the store.

- Oscar Mayer fat free bologna
- T. Marzetti fat free ranch and dill vegetable dips
- Fat Free Miracle Whip
- Kraft Fat Free Mayonnaise
- Raw Almonds (no salt added) (not fat free, but a handful is great for you at lunch)
- Any fat free cheese slices
- Any fat free bread
- Low fat or fat free turkey breast or chicken breast from your local deli
- All fat free crackers
- Fat free pudding cups and Jello cups
- All fruit cups (not in syrup and no added sugar!)
- All fat free hot dogs and fat free hot dog buns (yes, they're out there!)
- Fat free popcorn (hard to find…the low fat stuff isn't good enough and has too much salt)
- Grapes
- Strawberries, blueberries, or blackberries
- Fat free Pringles! (or any other fat free potato chips)
- Fat free Doritos!
- Fat free tortilla chips
- Fat free pretzels

Doesn't seem like much? That's because lunch is harder to find stuff for, yet it's easier in a way since you're limited by what you can pack anyway. When I show you my combinations next, you'll see what I mean. The following lunches can all fit into one zippered lunch container where ice packs fit in the bottom (which is what I use every day!), but remember, you can go as high in quantity as you wish.

If you want to bring a shopping bag full of food with you every day, go ahead! Just follow the no fat rule!

Also, I always would pack one can of diet pop with my lunch. Recently I started using one bottle of water instead. Use either one to suit your tastes.

1) Sandwich (or 2 or 3!) made of 2 fat free bologna slices and a slice or 2 of fat free cheese on 2 slices of fat free bread with either plain mustard or fat free Miracle Whip or both (with my ingredients, this sandwich is only 150 calories!). You can also substitute low fat turkey breast or low fat chicken breast, etc for the bologna, but the bologna is only 20 calories per slice and no fat! 1 cup of the yogurt. 1 cup of sugar free Jello or fat free pudding. Handful of almonds in a sandwich bag.

2) One of the above sandwiches. Cup of yogurt. Sandwich bag filled with baby carrots and/or sliced cucumbers (bring along a small cup of the fat free veggie dip). Sandwich bag filled with fresh strawberries.

3) One of the above sandwiches. Cup of yogurt. Baby carrots/cucumbers and dip. Handful of raw almonds in a sandwich bag. Cup of fat free pudding.

4) If you have microwave access, 2 fat free hot dogs in fat free buns. One bag of fat free microwave popcorn or as many fat free Pringles as you want. Cup of yogurt. Cup of sugar free Jello.

5) Baby carrots and dip. Fat free crackers and fat free cheese slices. Cup of yogurt. Handful of raw almonds. Sandwich bag full of grapes.

I could go on, but you're getting the idea now right? You can pack as much or as little as you want since usually, you've got to be quick at lunch time anyway. You'll get into the habit of packing this stuff at breakfast time, then bring the bag to and from work. It's easy, and it's a habit you will probably use for a very, very long time to come.

Now, just like your family and friends at home, your coworkers are not going to change, care about, or understand what you're doing. They'll try to convince you to order food with them or go to a pizza place for their all-you-can-eat lunch buffet. You are going to need to be ***vigilant!***

Just say NO! Once you start to lose a lot of weight, those people will respect you, but at first, whether they mean to or not, they'll try to thwart you every chance they get. I think this is secret jealousy at work since you have the willpower to better yourself and they don't. Whatever it may be, here's how you deal with it.

Remind yourself that you're in Stage 1 of The Logic Diet, and you can eat as much as you want and keep yourself full. Think about what you're going to have to eat when you get home and what your snacks will be tonight.

The stuff in your lunch bag is actually very good! You'll see that! Lastly, you'll feel a lot better the rest of the day since you didn't bog yourself down with a lot of melted cheese and such at lunch time. You'll see!

DINNER

Now you've made it through the day. You had your breakfast and lunch like you should, and since you're in Stage 1, you might have even had several snacks during the day already. It's now dinnertime, and you're in luck! I suggest that, in this Stage, you should definitely make this your biggest meal of the day.

Make sure you start the dinner process right when you get home. It may not be your style now, but you're going to have to make it a habit later, so you might as well start now. Remember, in Stage 1, you can eat more later if you want, so get dinner in you early!

Here is my list of dinner items. Again, have as much and as many different varieties of vegetables as you want. They are unlimited all throughout this diet plan. I will include my favorites in the list.

- Chicken breasts

- Top or bottom round steaks (NO other cuts of steak are allowed! They have too much fat)

- Lean burger patties (95/5 is preferred, but if you can't find them, 92/8 is acceptable. GO NO HIGHER!)

- Fat free hot dogs

- Fat free cheese slices

- Fat free *shredded* cheese (yes it's out there!)

- Any fat free refried beans

- Any fat free flour tortillas (yes they're out there too!)
- Any fat free salsa
- All fat free chips (tortilla or regular)
- All pasta (any kind, and have as much as you want in Stage 1)
- Any fat free pasta sauce (yes they make it!). Here I recommend Delallo Fat Free Marinara Sauce. I love this SO much, that I recommend going to Delallo.com and ordering it if you can't find it!
- Baked potatoes or yams (sweet potatoes are *wonderful* with spray butter!*)*
- Frozen vegetable blends
- Zucchini and zucchini squash
- Corn on the cob
- Canned vegetables (any kind you like)
- Any fat free butter spray (my favorite is Parkay)
- All fat free bread (and rolls and buns, etc if you can find them)
- Any fat free crackers
- All fat free salad dressings. My favorites here are Walden Farms Fat Free Sugar Free Calorie Free dressings (you heard me right!). Sound awful? Some of them taste FANTASTIC!! If you can't find them in the store, go to Waldenfarms.com and get them ordered. All the Italian varieties are my favorites. The Thousand Island, Jersey Sweet Onion, and Raspberry Vinaigrette are also great. I don't like any of the others. Their calorie free chocolate dip is also my favorite for use with strawberries! I do NOT recommend their pasta or barbeque sauces, but you can try for yourself of course!
- Shredded carrots
- Mushrooms
- Grape or cherry tomatoes
- Cucumbers

- Tilapia fish fillets

I'm going to stop here. There are many more foods out there you can find for dinner, so go ahead and mix it up. Also, later we'll get into snacks for those of you who can't live without food late at night. In Stage 1 it's OK!

Now before I get into some easy dinner combinations I use now and back when I was in Stage 1, I'm going to give you 2 of the many recipes I've come up with over the last couple years. I hope you like them!

Garlic Chicken Pasta

Ingredients:

- ½ package diced chicken breast pieces
- ½ cup Worcestershire sauce (if you can find Lea & Perrins for Chicken then even better)
- One can of fat free chicken broth
- 2 tbsp minced garlic OR garlic powder
- One package medium pasta shells (1 lb)
- One regular size bag of frozen vegetables (broccoli, cauliflower and water chestnuts are my favorite)
- One tbsp *brown* sugar (optional)
- ¼ cup fat free butter spray
- 1 tsp onion powder
- 1 tsp ground black pepper

Get a large wok and coat it with a non-stick, fat free, butter-flavored cooking spray. Combine Worcestershire sauce, chicken broth, garlic, brown sugar (if desired), butter spray (yes *pour it out*), onion powder, pepper, and diced chicken in the wok and set to medium heat. Stir every few minutes.

Start cooking your pasta as per the directions. Once your pasta has about 5 minutes left to cook, pour your frozen vegetables into the mixture in the wok (no need to defrost first) and stir to coat vegetables thoroughly. Stir the wok contents a couple times while the pasta finishes cooking.

Once pasta is to your desired tenderness, take off stove, drain pasta, and then dump pasta into the wok over everything else. Keep on medium heat and stir until you've got everything in there coated well with the broth mixture. It'll be a little tough to do with everything in there, so be careful and don't spill stuff everywhere!

Once coated well, leave on medium heat for just a couple more minutes to be sure vegetables are thoroughly cooked, then serve immediately in large bowls. I use a large strainer-serving spoon to put it into the bowls while removing some of the liquid, but it's not necessary.

Enjoy and eat as much as you want on Stage 1! Feel free to adjust recipe as you wish as long as you follow the rules!

Broiled Tilapia Fillets

<u>Ingredients:</u>

- 2 frozen Tilapia fillets per person you're cooking for

- Fat free butter spray

- Onion powder

- Garlic powder

- Ground black pepper

- Italian seasoning

Take your broiler pan and tray and cover the tray (with slots in it) with aluminum foil. Place back on top of the broiler pan, then use a knife to cut slits in the foil corresponding to the slots in the tray.

Place 4 frozen fish fillets on top of the foil (or 2 if it's just yourself.... OK 4 for just you if you're really hungry!). Spray coat fillets thoroughly with spray butter. Sprinkle or grind pepper lightly over fillets. Then coat the fillets *heavily* with the onion and garlic powders. Lastly, sprinkle a light coat of Italian seasoning on top.

Then flip the fillets over and repeat the same coatings on the other side.

Put in top rack of oven preheated to 400 degrees. Leave in to cook for 10 minutes, then flip the oven control to broil. Wait 3–5 minutes, then use a spatula (metal works best) to turn fillets over and broil 3–5 minutes on the other side. Be careful to watch closely so you don't burn them!

Serve and enjoy!

Now let's get to some of the dinner combinations I've used and how I make them. You can mix it up any way you'd like. I'm just trying to help get you started with some ideas! To drink, you should always have fat free sugar free liquids, such as water or diet pop. No sugary drinks!

1) Heat up some fat free refried beans, spread them on fat free flour tortillas, then cover with fat free shredded cheddar cheese, shredded lettuce, diced tomato, fat free sour cream, and taco sauce or salsa as you prefer. Roll up and heat for 30–60 seconds in the microwave and serve with fat free tortilla chips and salsa on the side. Add jalapeno peppers if desired. Have a Mexican style salad as well, with crushed fat free tortilla chips, etc. Or just have a regular salad with fat free dressing. I make mine with shredded carrots, grape tomatoes, and sliced mushrooms, sometimes with sliced cucumbers as well.

2) Cook 2 frozen chicken breasts on an indoor grill for about 8–10 minutes (no need to defrost!) or until thoroughly cooked. Cover with some fat free marinara sauce that you've heated in the microwave or on the stovetop. Serve with 1 or 2 baked potatoes with fat free butter spray and fat free sour cream. Have a small bowl of pasta and a salad on the side!

3) Do the same as above, but cover the chicken with barbeque sauce after cooked and serve with corn on the cob and a side of vegetables. I make my vegetables by taking a full bag of mixed veggies, usually broccoli and cauliflower mix, and pouring them into a microwave safe Tupperware container, pouring some fat free butter spray over the top, covering, and cooking for about 7–8 minutes. I then spray more butter on as needed while I eat them. Have a salad as well!

4) Try chicken Mexican style! After cooking as above, cover the chicken with some fat free shredded cheddar cheese and some of your favorite salsa, then

microwave for a minute to melt the cheese. Top with fat free sour cream (if desired). Serve with side of fat free tortilla chips and salsa and/or fat free flour tortillas filled with fat free refried beans. Don't forget your salad.

5) Cook 2 frozen lean burger patties the same as the chicken (again, no need to defrost before putting on your indoor grill!). Eat as you would a chopped steak with A-1 steak sauce (or your personal favorite). Serve with fat free bread slices and butter spray and have a potato or two as well. Salad of course.

6) Make 2 tilapia fillets as per my recipe. Serve with side of vegetables, fat free bread and butter spray, and salad.

7) Make my garlic chicken pasta and pig out on it! It's very filling, but you could still fit in some potatoes and salad on the side if you're really hungry.

8) Have a bottom round steak with 1 or 2 potatoes, bread and butter, and a salad on the side. Go ahead, have the vegetables too. You can eat as much of this stuff as you want!

9) Like the Mexican stuff from before? Try some nachos! Pile some fat free tortilla chips on an oven safe plate. Cover with fat free shredded cheeses, fat free refried beans (if desired), or even some lean ground beef (if desired). Bake in a preheated oven at 350 degrees for about 10 minutes. Serve with shredded lettuce, diced tomatoes, fat free sour cream, hot sauce and jalapenos (if desired), and salsa or your favorite taco sauce. Too bad I haven't found fat free taco shells yet, but if they make them, you can see what you could do here!

10) More chicken? After grilling, you can do many other things than what's listed above. Another one is to use a buffalo wing sauce or just *Tabasco* garlic or regular sauces to spice things up a bit. Mix up the sides as you wish.

11) Make some pasta the regular way. Serve with the fat free marinara sauce. For the side, take some fat free bread slices, cover with spray butter, then coat with some garlic salt and or garlic powder and maybe a little Italian seasoning, then bake in the oven at 350 degrees for about 5–8 minutes to make your own garlic bread. Have an Italian salad on the side. You won't notice the difference from your pasta nights before, and you'll be eating almost no fat!

As with the other meals, you can mix and match this up any way you want, and maybe have found other things that will work just as well for you that I haven't mentioned here.

Hopefully, you understand by now that you can do this! It takes a little work preparing your meals, but nobody said losing weight wouldn't be any work! Since you're able to eat this much food and stay full, it should feel very worth it to you to do this, because you'll see the weight coming off (you should start seeing results right away!).

Now you've eaten three big meals and you're watching your evening TV. Since you were always used to eating a lot of bad junk at night, you're getting hungry again. It may be because your brain is just used to it, or because you ate like a wooly mammoth before! Well, you're on Stage 1 for a reason, so remember, you can still eat at night! You will still see the weight come off!

You can eat anything you've been eating all day, again as long as its fat free, but I'll list some nighttime suggestions next that are a little less heavy and will prepare you better for the next Stages of the plan.

SNACKS

- Fat free potato chips, pretzels, or Doritos
- Fat free tortilla chips and salsa
- Fat free Jello cups
- Fat free pudding cups with fat free Cool Whip
- Grapes
- Strawberries and Walden Farms fat free chocolate dip (and the Cool Whip!)
- Baby carrots/cucumbers/sliced mushrooms and fat free vegetable dip
- Fat free hot dogs in fat free buns with ketchup, mustard and relish!
- Fat free grilled cheese sandwich. Toast 2 pieces of fat free bread, then coat insides of both pieces with spray butter and put in 2 slices of fat free sharp cheddar or American cheese. Put sandwich together and microwave for 20–30 seconds. AWESOME. (can use at lunch or dinner also!)
- Make a parfait using the fat free Cool Whip, fat free chocolate pudding, and mixed berries

- Fat free yogurt cups

- Flavored coffee with fat free creamer and calorie free sweetener

- Make the fat free nachos or burritos I described earlier

- Fat free crackers and fat free cheese slices

- Reduced fat vanilla wafers or wheat thins (just be careful to stay under the day's fat gram allowance)

- Any fat free cookies, cakes or the like you can find

- Fat free angel food cake (great with strawberries!)

There are going to be a lot more and all kinds of variations based on what you find out there. The best thing is the flexibility you'll have as your mind and body gets through the adjustment to the new plan you're embarking on.

CHEATING ON STAGE 1

Now as I wrote earlier, I **_FORBID_** cheating on Stage 1! You have too much flexibility of what you can eat and when you can eat it to do that. By cheating, I mean going off altogether and eating fattening foods of any kind. I don't care how hard you think it is! You are losing weight while eating all day! If you're hungry, you can eat! Just NOT the bad stuff. PERIOD!

The reason behind this is that, once you are through Stage 1, there are going to be times I let you cheat, because it gets much harder and you'll need to be able to reward yourself sometimes. Also, I want your mind and body to get used to the idea that those old, bad foods you used to indulge in are no longer going to be on the menu. My plan lets you stay full so you gradually do this! Remember that no other plan allows for that! So…NO CHEATING DURING STAGE 1!

DOES STAGE 1 HAVE TO END?

Unfortunately, it does. You're probably asking when and how. The when is going to be entirely subjective based on your body and how overweight you were when you started. Mine lasted about 3 months, but I think many of you will be on it for a shorter time than that. The only real way to tell that Stage 1 is over is simple enough. It's when you stop losing weight!

Now you have to be sure your body isn't just on a plateau. A plateau, as I use the term here, is when your weight sticks at an exact amount for at least 1 week without dropping at all. Once you're up to 2 weeks, it's not a plateau anymore. At that point, you need to move to Stage 2. I like to give it a full 2 weeks just to be sure.

There will be some plateaus that will last less than 2 weeks while you're on Stage 1. It's important to be vigilant during these times. Don't jump ahead in the plan too quickly, and certainly don't give up and go off the diet thinking it isn't working since you haven't lost an ounce in a week. Just know you're on a plateau and that it's natural as your body adjusts to the changes you're making in your lifestyle. I'll talk more about plateaus later.

At this point in this discussion, I'll give you my thought on when and how often you should weigh yourself. A lot of material I've read and heard about out there says you shouldn't weigh yourself every day since there are all kinds of natural fluctuations in the body and your weight can fluctuate by as much as 5 pounds per day, etc. This holds true for people eating normally who don't have to diet much. For my plan, I am in disagreement here!

On The Logic Diet, you should definitely weigh yourself every single day, and it must be at the exact same time, if at all possible, every single day! It must be before you start eating for the day, no matter when you wake up, and cannot be right after any meal or snack.

I weigh myself at 7:00 am every single morning. I say this because, on my plan, you will always be on a path where you will be seeing results in your weight loss. If you aren't checking on it daily, you might miss a sign that things are going wrong or that you need to move to the next stage. Since there's no way your weight should be going *up* if you aren't cheating, it will not hurt to do it daily. Lastly, the boost in your willpower will increase a ton when you're seeing results more often than once per week!

Now you don't have to read on to the next Stage if you're working on Stage 1. Just keep losing the weight until the plateaus are all over and you've maintained for 2 weeks at the same weight level.

I've thought back to when I was finished with Stage 1. I remember how great I felt. I hadn't eaten fast food for months, I had lost over 25 pounds and gone down 2 pant sizes already. I was used to eating three meals per day and was finding great snacks to keep me full when I had cravings. Here's where I would have been in trouble had I not set that original goal. I was at about 243 lbs and holding, and had a fleeting thought that I could just stay like that!

Remember the reasons that motivated you to do this in the first place. I still couldn't run and play like I wanted to. My son had just turned 2 years old and I knew I had to get much lower and start moving around more if I was going to be his sports mentor. So I forged ahead.

I knew what I had to do next, I just wasn't looking forward to it. So I now present you with what I consider to be the hardest Stage of this plan, at least when it comes to willpower. Other parts of the diet may require more thought and planning, but this part is all about willpower and control.

So gather yourself…be prepared to lose a bunch more weight…and read ahead.

Stage 2

No More Eating Late

That by itself sounds just terrible, doesn't it? Well that's just too bad. On this plan, you have no choice but to do it. That's why I start this now. You'll still be able to eat what you want (following the fat gram rule of course) and how much you want. Now you'll just have to control the ***when*** part.

I know you've been used to eating during your late night TV shows and during those nighttime movie sessions with your friends or family, but it is part of what's causing you to be overweight and it needs to end!

If you think it doesn't matter that you eat late as long as you're eating better foods, you're wrong. You've heard the one about how eating right before bedtime giving you nightmares. That's closer to the truth. The nightmare is how what you eat at night sticks to your body and becomes part of all of that fat you're trying to get rid of.

If you're serious…truly serious about losing the weight and keeping it off forever, then you'll accept this step and put your willpower to the test in order to accomplish it. Those out there that are already thin DO NOT eat *anything*, let alone junk food, late at night or before bedtime.

There's a reason for that. It's a reason you haven't cared about before. Now you care, and you're going to take the steps necessary to eliminate this bad habit.

Now we'll discuss the definition of "late" as it relates to my plan.

WHAT IS LATE?

This would be easy if everyone in the world was on the same daily schedule, but I'm painfully aware that isn't the case.

For those of you on what I call the "regular" work schedule, which I would define as starting anywhere from 6:30–8:00 AM and ending anywhere from 3:00–5:30 PM (I fall into this category), late refers to 7:00 PM. That means **NO EATING AFTER 7:00 PM!**

Of course many of you aren't on that "regular" schedule. Some of you may even blame your abnormal schedule, at least in part, for causing you to be more overweight.

I'm telling you now that it makes no difference *what* your schedule is. You still can have 3 meals per day at certain intervals, and you can stop eating after a certain point during *your* day.

For those of you on the abnormal work schedule, I will set the rule in these terms. You must have breakfast after you get up in the morning and before you go to work, and you must stop eating a minimum of 3 hours before you go to bed, whenever that may be. I prefer at least 4 hours, but 3 will be good enough.

I will answer the questions as to why soon enough. For now just understand this is going to be a steadfast rule of this plan and you must follow it no matter what! I will let you know later what to do if you think you can't handle it!

Now let's get back to those on the normal schedule. Don't read the above paragraph and think that means you can eat at 9:00 since you're going to bed at midnight. For you, the rule is steadfast. 7:00 PM is the cutoff. ***PERIOD!***

THE LOGIC BEHIND STAGE 2

So, as you're thinking about the above statements in terror, you're wondering why this is necessary. There are some theories and articles out there that would tell you that this doesn't matter. They would tell you that the amount of calories you eat in a day is what it is, and it doesn't matter when they are consumed. To me, this is an unbelievable falsehood, and will stop you from reaching your goals and being satisfied with yourself in the future.

Here's the main reason why. Like I said earlier, weight is lost by reducing the calories you eat in relation to the calories **you burn** throughout the day. If you eat late at night or right before bedtime, you will not be burning those calories off any more that day! Your metabolism slows down when you sleep, and those calories you eat late at night just sit there and turn into unwanted pounds and body fat. Yes, I've read you can burn calories while you sleep, but I've never seen it work.

What I *did* see work was when I stopped eating late, I lost another 20 pounds in a very short time (about 2 months). The simple fact is that you're cutting off a portion of the day where you're able to eat, and therefore eating fewer calories as a result. This, coupled with the fact that you're burning the calories you have eaten that day for a longer time, will make you lose weight.

Remember, everything I have you do is to gradually lead you into the way of life when you'll be thinner and healthier. This step makes sense for a few reasons. You get out of the habit of eating junk food while watching late night TV and movies. You get into the habit of eating a good-sized, healthy dinner after you get home from work. You give yourself more energy at night to pursue other fun nighttime activities.

You'll be happy that you've gotten used to eating those great breakfasts now! You'll go to bed a little hungrier, but wake up refreshed and ready to eat your energy and metabolism-boosting meal to start off the day.

Skipping the late night food will also keep you feeling less bogged down at night. You'll be amazed at how great you'll feel. It will just take awhile for your brain to get used to the idea. So read on.

TRICKS OF THE TRADE

OK, so you've gotten your mind ready, your willpower strengthened, and your resolve intact. You're going to make this work, and you're committed to following this plan until you're at your goal weight (or lower!). Good for you! But…UH, OH…your body is sitting there at 9:30 PM and making your mind turn twists in your head.

You think there's no way you're going to make it if you don't eat, and of course, your mind is saying that, if you're going to go off the diet, it might as well be with fudge cake!

I'll help you not allow this to happen! And if it does, I'll help you get through it. You have to understand that you have conditioned yourself to be the overweight person you are. More than likely, you've been eating late your whole life, and the foods you were eating late were probably the worst foods you were eating all day.

It's very hard for your mind to get used to the idea that you can watch TV at night without munching or crunching on something. It's almost as hard as quitting smoking in my opinion, so you definitely need help with this one. I believe that only on my plan can you have it as easy as you do the rest of the day while you're trying to wean yourself off of late-night eating at this stage of the game.

So for those of you that don't think you can make it, I'm going to give you the tips and tricks you'll need in order to complete this most-important step toward improving your looks and your health.

EAT DINNER RIGHT BEFORE YOUR TIME DEADLINE

Sounds so simple, so why aren't you doing it! On this plan, it makes the most sense, and makes it the easiest on you, if you start cooking your dinner around 6:15 to 6:30 so you'll be done right at or about 7:00. Of course, those of you on the abnormal schedules can adjust this to about an hour before your particular cutoff time.

When I first started Stage 2, I thought to myself "OK…if I can't eat past 7:00, I'm going to eat right up until that clock ticks it!" That's exactly what I did. I started to get into the habit of starting dinner preparations right when I got home from work, which was right about 5:30–6:00 PM. If I had to take care of my 2 children that night, since my wife is a nurse and works a lot of night shifts, I'd start their dinner then as well.

If I got home from work later than usual due to problems or late customers at work, I'd prepare the faster and easier of my menu items or include lots of ready-made fat free stuff that was quicker to serve.

You see, I understand that you have a busy life. You have work schedules that aren't always the exact same every day. You have children and spouses that can throw off your schedule. I'm here to tell you that you can work around this, you *must* work around this, if you're going to succeed long term.

Again, you're changing your entire *lifestyle* here, not just what you're eating. You have to make that commitment and stick with it! You should expect those around you to accommodate you to help you reach your goal. If they don't, then you'll have to do it in spite of them!

Now, if circumstances arise to where you absolutely, positively cannot start dinner prior to your cutoff time, then just go ahead and make it as soon as you possibly can after that point. I should hope this happens to you no more than once every couple weeks if you're an extremely busy person or have one of those crazy jobs where you work 80 hours a week or something like that.

I am NOT advocating skipping dinner altogether if you're going to be late. Skipping meals will only hurt you in the long run and will foil your attempt to lose weight properly.

Anyway, if you're making your dinner and eating it right before the cutoff, you'll have a better chance of making it through the night without going crazy and cheating. If it's still hard, then have an extra large dinner right before cutoff!

Remember, during *this* Stage, you can still eat ***as much*** as you want of the fat free and low fat stuff, so **pig out** at dinner.

Have 3 chicken breasts and 3 baked potatoes if it'll help! Have a whole pound of pasta and fat free sauce! Eat the entire portion of my garlic chicken pasta all by yourself (I've done that many times)!

What other plan would allow you to do this and still claim it'll help you lose weight? NONE OF THEM! Be thankful, as I was, that you can adjust to all of this in this manner. When I absolutely stuffed myself at dinner, even if it was with extra vegetables, it just made everything that much easier!

All right, so you've done all of this and you just still can't make it. You're new to Stage 2 and you used to eat so much at night that your brain can't take it no matter how much you're eating at dinner. Well my plan aims to please and make it easy for you to change, so here goes.

Acceptable Snacks If You're Going To Crack

If you absolutely can't make it, and your brain's telling you to go for your kids' fudge cake at 10:00 PM, there are things you can eat to take the edge off and only cause extremely minimal damage to the plan and your psyche. If you're serious about this plan, you will cause yourself major guilt and have a hard time dealing mentally with the next day if you cheat at night, so use my snacks only.

Before I get into it, I'm telling you now that these are not to become nighttime allowances that you eat every night because you're still seeing weight loss results. You need to change your brain so your lifestyle transformation will be a permanent one.

These are for emergencies only. These are for those times when you feel that if you don't eat something you're just going to scrap the whole thing because you're just not mentally tough enough.

It's OK to think that way sometimes. Remind yourself that it's normal. It's VERY hard to do what you're doing. Most of us had been in the bad habits of eating our entire lives. Those are major tendencies and habits to break!

The difference now is that you have guidelines to help change you, and the plan you're on helps you do it gradually!

OK, here's the *emergency only* nighttime list. I wouldn't deviate from this at all, since these are the only ones I found for myself that worked. The list is short…sorry!

- Baby carrots, mushrooms, or cucumbers and fat free vegetable dip
- Sugar free Jello cups (only 10 calories each, so have a few!)
- Grapes (don't go crazy!)
- Flavored coffee with fat free creamer and sugar substitute

Don't knock the coffee until you've tried it. Any calorie free liquids are free at night, and the coffee, while having a few calories, can make you feel like you're having a chocolate treat (or cinnamon or vanilla, etc) while filling you up well if you have 2 large cups of it. Can't have caffeine at night? Use decaf!

- Strawberries, blueberries, raspberries, or blackberries and fat free or sugar free Cool Whip (and/or Walden Farms Calorie Free Chocolate Dip!) (have a couple pints of berries if you want)

- One sugar free or fat free pudding cup topped with Cool Whip

That's it. The list is short, and it should be! Many nights when I was on Stage 2, I would have strawberries and the dip, or 2 large cups of coffee, and it would get me through the craving period very easily. Other times, if the cravings weren't as bad, I'd just have an extra large plastic cup filled with Diet Coke (or my favorite diet pop), and I'd be fine!

To give you a taste of the future, I'll fill you in a little bit on how my life is now. At this point, I can eat dinner at 4:30 if I wanted to (if I'm home early or on the weekends) and still not eat anything the rest of the night. I have no cravings at night at all, and do not eat anything while watching my late night TV. My brain is totally conditioned to not eat at night, and it got that way during Stages 2 and 3.

CHEATING ON STAGE 2

As you know, I didn't let you cheat at all during Stage 1. That doesn't apply anymore. If you've been stringent, and kept your willpower high, you've now been on my plan probably between 2–4 months and have already lost between 20 and 40 pounds (maybe even more if you were more than 100 pounds overweight when you started Stage 1). So now you've got something to celebrate, and you also have to learn a few things about cheating and what your body will do with those old, bad foods you used to eat all day.

Cheating here is not regimented or planned out for you. You'll know when it's time to cheat for the first time on this plan. Your mind will tell you one day. You can also plan it out for an important occasion such as an anniversary or birthday, or maybe a big family gathering on a holiday. Whatever the reason may be, here is how you're going to cheat on this plan.

EAT WHATEVER YOU WANT, ALL DAY AND ALL NIGHT. You heard me right! When you cheat on my plan, at least during this Stage, you are really going to cheat. Don't hold yourself back. Let your mind take a break from the stress. Get up in the morning, go to IHOP, pig out, go to Taco Bell for lunch, and go out for dinner as well!

Get a pie or cake from the market and eat the whole thing at 10:30 PM if you want! Eat *Snickers* bars all day in between meals. I want you to **really** reward yourself for a whole day when you cheat, so that you have no regrets about that day off. You're going to say to yourself, "That was worth it."

Now, you can call me crazy, but if you were really big like I was, and started at Stage 1 like I did, you'll understand why this way of cheating is so great and rewarding. You'll also notice that you'll be able to eat just like you did before, which is an unfortunate side effect of our prior lifestyles that, I'm sorry to say, still has not gone away from me as much as I'd like even to this day. I can still almost pack the food away when I want to just like I did when I was 268 lbs.

Anyway, I'm allowing you to do this for one day and one day only the first time you cheat. You're not ready for more than that yet, so make that day count, and make sure you're not setting yourself up to make it more than one day if you can help it at all.

I understand that, depending on when you start my plan, Christmas or Thanksgiving may be in the mix, and family vacations always cause a problem. During my early Stages, I say go ahead and take off in full for a family vacation as well as the major holidays. You understand by now that this plan is going to be a long process, so skipping a few days, or even a week for a vacation, is *not* going to matter in the long term.

Otherwise, stick to one day only. You'll find that this helps your mind, and also will actually help your body! Other than the short term effects you'll notice (like running to the bathroom a lot…boy, those bad foods really tear you up!), cheating for a day will trick your metabolism a little, and help you shake things up with your body so that the plan will kick in quicker and more effectively the week after.

The next morning after a cheat day, you are to get up, take your supplements, and start breakfast just as you did before the cheat day. You're not going to want to eat in the morning, but you must do it! Do **not** let one day off change your newly formed habits even once!

You need that breakfast in order to start your metabolism off right for that day, even if your belly still feels full from the night before. Don't worry, your body will get rid of that prior day's feasting soon enough (probably right after your breakfast)!

At this point, I want to tell you about what the cheating is going to mean to you as far as how much of a setback it will be. Many of you want to have everything metered out in detail, and I am like that as well. So lucky for you, I analyzed everything I did and what effect it had on me and my weight loss plan.

THE MATH OF CHEATING

Here is how the cheating on my plan is going to effect the plan itself. Assuming you're following the plan as it has been laid out for you, you can expect the following:

1. For every full day off you take, it will take 3 full days on my plan to get back to the weight you were before the day off. This is exact! So, if you take 4 days off in a row, it will take you 12 days to get back. 10 days = 30! I'm dead serious! It works to the day!

2. If you take a half-day off, it depends on when (and this is more proof to me that eating at night is a bad thing!). If you take the first half of a day off **only**, then it will only take you 1 full day to get back to the weight prior! If you take the latter half of a day off, it will ***still take you 3 days to get back!*** I've tested this many times, and it holds true!

Now, I haven't started talking about cheating only for one meal, or having a dessert one day, or anything like that. We're only in Stage 2, and that's talk for Stages 5 and 6, so don't get ahead of yourself, and don't change things up. Remember, I'm setting your mind up for a gradual life change. Don't speed it up, or your mind may let you down!

So even when you cheat for only half a day, make it worth it! Eat as much as you want during that time! I've done a greasy spoon breakfast, burgers for lunch, then my plan's dinner, and got back to my weight after one day back on the plan. If cheating at night is more your thing, then I suggest just making it a whole day, since it will still take 3 days to get back.

Talk about logic! I love rationalizing things like that, especially if it means I can eat a strawberry covered cheesecake at 10:00 PM on my day off!

WHEN DOES STAGE 2 END?

So when do you move to the next Stage? Similar to Stage 1, this should end whenever you stop losing weight for at least 2 weeks. However, I would suggest staying on this Stage as long as you need to in order to break your late night snacking habits.

If you're using my snacks too often even after your weight-loss plateaus have ended, you should stay on this Stage until you're totally comfortable with not eating after dinner and are no longer relying on the snack list to help get you through that.

Look, we're not on the lose 10 pounds in 10 days mindset here! You're really changing yourself, so give it time! If you've been following my plan to the letter up to this point, you're already comfortable with this idea, so truly stay on this Stage until you can handle the next step!

Stage 3 is where it starts to get a little more difficult and you ***need*** to be mentally ready in order to handle it properly.

Don't read ahead in this book either if you can help it. You are supposed to be doing this gradually and making sure each Stage sticks permanently before you move along. I know you're curious about what comes next and you're also not used to stopping and starting a book in that manner.

Understand again that I completed this plan over about a year and a half! I will say that I did have an idea of what I was going to do next (until Stage 5 that is), but I tried not to think ahead so I would finish each step fully before I tried the next.

Stage 3

Reduce Portions

You've made it very far now on your way to a new body. Congratulations! You've passed Stages 1 and 2, and have probably lost over 40 pounds by now, and maybe a lot more! You're still a long way from your goal, however, and it's time to start getting serious about getting closer to that goal.

So, if you're ready to go with the next step, then you should not have lost any weight in at least the last two weeks, and should not be eating at night at all anymore, not even my snacks.

If that's the case, then you're definitely ready. I say this is an easy Stage for you, but some minds may find it a lot more difficult than I did. You see, I had the problem giving up late night eating, but you may find it harder to finally cut down on **how much** you've been eating.

That is rule #1 for Stage 3. You must reduce your portions at every meal, and cut out the snacks (yes, even the fat free ones) in between meals, so that you're left eating 3 meals per day ***only***.

This will not be easy. The simplest way for me to explain how to do this is to say for you to go ahead and just cut your meals in half at each meal, as well as cutting out all the daytime snacking. I do not know, however, how much you've decided to eat at each meal, so, in your case, you may have to cut breakfast and dinner in half, but leave lunch the same since it was already just a fat-free cheese sandwich and a cup of yogurt.

If your dinner includes 2 of anything, just make it 1 instead, like potatoes, burger patties, or chicken breasts. If you were having 2 ears of corn, make it one. Leave your salad there as before, and you can always have your vegetable mixture every night.

At breakfast, if you were eating 4 pieces of fat free toast, make it 2. It you were having 2 egg-substitute sandwiches, make it 1, and so on. Since I advocate 3 servings of yogurt per day, you can still have 2 for breakfast, or make it 1 at each meal, however you want to do it.

You're getting the point. You will be consuming much less food each day now, and will definitely start getting hungrier because of it. Now your mind is ready for this step though!

Other diet plans have you starting out here or include this with the first part of their plans. The plans that ship the food to your door are basically based on this principle of portion control! Imagine starting one of those plans before Stage 1! Think about that as you start this Stage.

I've given you months of preparation before you have to do this! It worked like a charm for me. By this point, I was so looking forward to seeing the weight drop even further, and had been getting so motivated by the results I was seeing weekly thus far, that it was easy for me to cut back so I could keep the show rolling and the pants size shrinking!

There is also a rule #2 for Stage 3. That is the following: YOU NOW MUST ALSO CUT OUT AS MUCH SUGAR AND SALT (SODIUM) AS POSSIBLE FROM THE FAT FREE AND LOW FAT FOODS YOU'RE CONSUMING.

I could have instituted this rule right at Stage 1, or rolled it out in Stage 2. Maybe you're already at the low point of these 2 things, but probably not. This means that, if you have still been using that saltshaker at the dinner table (or any other time), it stops NOW. If you have been using a lot of fat free foods that have high sugar contents to get you by, those must now GO.

You will still get enough sodium for your daily diet through the foods you're eating, trust me. Excess salt in your system just holds in water weight, and when you cut it out, you'll see those pounds fall off. The excess sugar just adds excess calories, and as we move to Stage 4, you'll be focusing on those calories every day, so you're cutting out the sugar now to let yourself down more easily to that next level.

This is a RULE folks! It is REQUIRED. Just keep trusting me and DO IT! If it means no more fat free fruit snacks, then you'll just have to live with it. You won't be able to eat those later anyway so trust me!

THE LOGIC BEHIND STAGE 3

As I've said a few times already during this book, and will surely say again at some points forward, you lose weight as a direct result of reducing the calories you consume in comparison to the calories you are burning per day. This Stage is simply reducing your calories without making you bury yourself in the details yet.

I'll leave that for Stage 4. The main logic behind my plan (again as I've said a few times already!) is to bring you down *gradually* so that the weight loss will stick and your mind can handle the life-long transition. I believe that if you try to get to the end too fast, you'll end up giving up and gaining all the weight back.

So this is the easy way to cut calories without having to think too much about it. In the first 2 Stages, you've been able to eat as **much** as you want, just controlling first *what* you're eating, then second *when* you're eating it.

Now you are finally starting to control the *how much* part, just easing into it instead of going hard core like most other diet plans would have you do.

Portions truly are the devil when it comes to how much you weigh. Think about when you went out to restaurants before. If the portions weren't huge, you complained that you weren't getting enough for your money. This is why most restaurants out there serve such massive portions!

The thin people leave more than half their food on the plate and have no room for dessert. The overweight people are the ones you see finishing all of the food and waiting there for another half hour in order to be ready to eat the excessively large dessert as well! I used to be like that, and many of you were as well.

It's interesting that the "joke" about the really expensive restaurants you go to only on special occasions (or more often if you're rich!) is that you pay all that money and the portions are tiny! These restaurants understand that it's the quality of the food, not the quantity, that should be important, and that the people out there that care about their bodies eat based on a calorie intake of normal proportions.

Anyway, up until now, you've probably been using fat free snacks during the day to help you make it until the next meal time, then having that huge meal right before 7:00 to get you though the night.

Now that you'll be cutting those snacks out and reducing the size of those meals, as well as getting rid of the extra salt and sugar, you'll understand what I said earlier about how you'll be *loving* some of those foods you've found. You'll be ***looking forward*** to all 3 of your meals, because you really do love them!

Before I started this plan, I never thought I'd be looking forward to eating a microwave container full of broccoli, cauliflower, and sliced green and yellow zucchini squash covered in spray butter, but now I can't wait to get my fork into it at dinner time!

You took food for granted before (especially the fatty, greasy kind). Now you'll appreciate the better, healthier foods that you'll be consuming more of for the rest of your life.

By this time, several months have gone by, if not longer, and your body has gotten rid of those cravings for the bad foods. You're already feeling healthier and stronger. You have more energy than you've had in years, and you've dropped several (if not more!) pant sizes.

What's more logical than all of this!

QUANTIFYING STAGE 3

So. You're asking…How much will I lose in this Stage? How long will it take? How diligent do I have to be? How do I measure what I'm cutting back?

The answers to all of these questions are subjective. You are most likely doing this plan a little differently than I did, and differently than anyone else is doing it. Sticking to my rules is a must, but there are many ways to do this. Measuring what you cut back on should not be a chore in math. Again, wait until later. You'll have to do plenty of that soon enough! Just follow what I said before about cutting back at each meal and all mid-day snacks. It'll be enough! Trust me!!

How much you will lose will depend a lot on how big you were to start with. If you were like me, you'll still be able to lose between 10 and 20 pounds on this Stage. You may lose a lot more if you were really big, but that means this Stage will be harder and longer for you. If you were not as big as me, you may lose only 5–10 pounds and this Stage may be very short.

Remember, it's important to go through it for your *mind*. You are transitioning yourself into your final lifestyle. So take as long as you want on this Stage. You do have to be diligent and consistent though in what you're cutting back on. You can't have 1 burger patty today, then go back to 2 tomorrow. You can't eliminate your mid-day snack today, then have it again tomorrow. You must be consistent every single day! If you could make it through Stage 2, this should be easy for you!

CHEATING ON STAGE 3

Cheating on this Stage does NOT mean you can have a snack in between meals or go back to a bigger portion meal on a certain day. You must not do this at all costs!

You are staying consistent with the plan every day, and cheating in that way would cause you to lose that consistency.

Cheating in this Stage is the exact same as it was in Stage 2! If you're going to go off for a day or two (or a week's vacation!), then GO OFF. Eat your face off for the day, or half of the day, whatever you decide. Remember how much it will set you back as regards your final weight goal. Then, the day after the carnage, go right back to the plan and the smaller portions per meal you were using the day before you went off!

Your mind is well equipped now to handle these days off with flair, knowing you'll be right back on the plan the next day and right back past your pre-cheat weight in a few days.

You might even be getting sick and tired of eating the bad foods on your cheat days already! You'll feel a little yucky the day after, and you'll start to understand a little better how the other half have always been able to avoid eating like you used to.

You don't feel good after you eat them! But if you're not over them yet, don't worry about it AT ALL. I've NEVER gotten over some of it! To me, Taco Bell will always be the food of the gods! (and Cold Stone Creamery is the dessert of the gods...)

Remember though that these days should not be taken too often. If you feel you're going to crack, or you're going on a vacation, then fine, but otherwise you should be resisting temptation to go off the plan as hard as you possibly can. Remember, you *are* on a diet after all! You can't cheat a whole bunch and expect it to work!

We're only going to start changing how the cheating works starting in Stage 5. So you do have a lot more cheat days to look forward to for a long time! During this Stage, I started using those days as a reward. I would pick a date a few weeks ahead, or know I had an occasion coming up with family or friends that I would like to be able to eat during, then look forward with high anticipation to that day, and sometimes plan out exactly what I would eat in advance!

There's nothing wrong with rewarding yourself! You're working very hard at this and showing great results. Nobody thought you could do it. Don't worry that people will think you're going to gain all the weight back when they see you pigging out on a reward day. Let them think that way!

You know you've got the plan to go back to the next day, and you know that it's ***foolproof***. You've seen by now that it works exactly like I said it would, so that confidence in the results you're getting each week will give you the strength to do these cheat days and know you'll have no problem going back to the plan the next day. You'll see!

What other plan out there gives you this kind of opportunity! Where else could you pig out on burgers and fries all day and have a huge ice-cream sundae at 11:00 that night (I used to do that!), and still promise weight loss if you stick to the plan! Remember you're on the greatest plan out there, so be happy with it!

WHEN DOES STAGE 3 END (AND DOES IT HAVE TO)?

Now we come to an interesting quandary. You've maintained the plan exactly as you were supposed to. You have passed your weight plateau test at this Stage, and now should be moving on. Before we say anything else, remember, you can stay at this Stage as long as you want to keep your mind healthy. If you don't feel you can handle what's coming next, then don't start yet.

The quandary is this…some of you have lost over 50 pounds already. I was at about that, weighing in at 220 pounds. My original goal weight had been 215 pounds, so I was almost already there. If you set your goal as we discussed in that section, you should still have a little way to go (or a lot), but some of you are looking in the mirror, as I did at this point, and thinking to yourself it might not be that terrible if I just continued at Stage 3 forever!

You're thinking that you're looking and feeling better than you have in years, and many people are telling you how great you look as well!

You're saying to yourself that it's really easy to eat like you're eating. Maybe it's not worth the stress of going further. Maybe you don't feel like it's worth pushing yourself any more to lose another 10–20 pounds (some of you may still need to lose a lot more than that so disregard this!). Maybe you feel you could just use Stage 3 as a maintenance diet for the rest of your days.

It's true that I think you could succeed in doing this. It would work and you might even be very happy keeping things right where they are now. You could always try it out for awhile…keep doing Stage 3 for a few more months maintaining at the weight you are and taking cheat days as you need them, etc…then pick up where you left off later if you decide you want to lose more weight.

I'll say this…I didn't feel complete at this point. I loved the smaller clothes and all the positive compliments I was getting, but I just felt like I was falling short. My mind told me that I wasn't quite where I should be, and that it felt like people were getting a little jealous. Maybe they secretly didn't want me to keep going…maybe they didn't want me to get thinner and healthier then they were…?

Whatever the reason I did it, I'm sure glad I kept going. This is when I created a new goal for myself of 205 pounds and came up with the next Stage in my plan so I could get there. Of course, I ended up getting even further, I just didn't know I could yet.

I'll say that the next steps truly work. This is where a lot of people—those looking for a way to lose vanity pounds or to finish off where another diet plan they were on failed them—are going to *start* my plan.

Perhaps you can say that you are on par with those people now! Maybe you are someone who most people would consider healthy and in a relatively good weight range! Maybe you are someone who's just looking to lose that extra 10–30 pounds like everyone else! Doesn't that feel great!!

If you were extremely overweight to start with and you don't feel these comments relate to you, then you can disregard them. You're headed in the right direction and everyone knows it. Just keep focused and stay on this Stage until you're mentally ready for the next.

For the rest of you I say go forward. Don't stop now. You've done great things, and you can handle what's coming next. It will give you great knowledge that you can use for the rest of your life to maintain the new body you're creating, and will create habits you won't break in the future.

GEARING UP FOR STAGE 4

So you've decided to go forward and get to the last weight loss Stage you'll need to get to your goal (or beyond!). Congratulations! This is going to be the most rewarding Stage of this plan!

It will, however, also be the most work. It will take planning, some research, and strict execution for it to work as laid out on these pages. That doesn't mean you will need to be a rocket scientist or a mathematician in order to do this. I will spell it out for you and help you through it every step of the way.

Just make sure that your mind is ready to proceed. The best way to know you're ready is if you're having such an easy, comfortable time on Stage 3 that you don't even consider it a slight problem anymore to be on the plan. It should be second nature by now. Maybe you've even thrown in a little exercise (or a lot if you're into that) and have seen the results come even quicker than most.

You also need to still be a little, or a lot, dissatisfied with your weight or how you look. Maybe you still want to get to a certain size of clothing or want a more toned look to your upper body. Maybe it's just as simple as that scale and what the number shows.

Whatever the reason, it needs to be enough to push you past the easiness of where you've been thus far, and into the difficulty of monitoring yourself like you're going to need to.

I'm here to tell you that you can do this. If I did it, anyone can. The trick was teaching myself *how* to do it, which you don't have to go through because I'm going to tell you the how!

So with that taken out of it, I'm sure you can accomplish this part, and make it to wherever you want or need to be to make yourself happy. You'll continue to be very healthy as well I promise!

So steel yourself. Tell yourself that you *are* ready. Believe that it will still be easy for you. Finally, get ready to help yourself get to the weight you've dreamed of being at for a very long time.

Stage 4

Counting Calories (The Right Way)

Welcome to the nitty-gritty. Here we are at the most demanding Stage of this plan. For those of you who are new to my plan altogether and are just starting right here at Stage 4, welcome! You are that person who is smaller to begin with that my other readers. Or perhaps you are the female reader who is naturally a smaller body type, but is only 15–40 pounds overweight.

Maybe you're the one who just can't seem to lose those extra 10 pounds left over from your other dieting efforts. Well, unless you have a biological issue or have some other problem losing weight where you need a doctors input, I'd say that no matter what your other plan or situation was, this ***will*** work for you!

For the rest of you, congratulations for making it this far. By now, you've been on my plan for anywhere from 4–8 months and have probably lost anywhere from 40–80 pounds or more! You have been led down the path of changing your entire lifestyle in a slow, well-metered manner, and you have succeeded! Now you just want to finish the job. You want to get to that final goal, or get to that last clothing size you've always wanted to attain, or had attained a long, long time ago.

For those of you who have been with me since the beginning, I'm going to remind you now that, if you haven't been taking the supplements I recommended to you at Stage 1, you are now REQUIRED to take them.

For those of you just starting with me, I will list them again here. You must take a daily multivitamin (whichever you choose) and 1000 mg of Calcium fortified with 400 IU of Vitamin D. I still take 1000 mg of Vitamin C, but it's not required (and my doctor said it's unnecessary). You could also start taking the 500 mg of cinnamon in tablet form if you wish. I'm still not convinced it does anything though.

As alluded to at the end of the last Stage, and in the title of this Stage, you're going to be counting calories, and I mean counting them *exactly*. Now I've read many times in many places that a lot of people out there don't want to count calories because it's too much work or because they don't have the time.

Well, those of you who have been through my entire plan should be happy to do it because, a few months ago, you would've done anything to look like you do now, and you have the confidence in what's going on to take the last step toward your dreams.

The rest of you reading here have tried those other methods that stayed away from calorie counting **_and they didn't work for you_**. So, naturally, you should be OK with this as well.

I will say it *again* (and again and again if necessary), and many other texts and articles out there will echo this statement: Weight is lost in the relationship between how many calories you take in during the day and how many calories you burn during the day.

If you want to do this right, and make it absolutely *foolproof*, then you must **track** *exactly* how many calories you are taking in! I will provide you with the number to judge this against so don't worry.

The math of it is the easy part. It's the tracking that's the hard part. That's what I'm going to teach you all to do in this Stage of the plan. As I say in the title, we're going to do this the right way, and there is only one right way as far as I'm concerned. It will take a lot of work at first, but gets much easier as you go forward, since you'll most likely be putting it all on paper for you to keep as your own personal reference guide.

Make no mistake; your guide will be specific to you and only you. You cannot find a guide out there that you can use. You will have to create your own!

Are you ready yet? Well here we go!

THE RESULTS ARE IN THE MATH

For you to be able to lose weight in this Stage, you need to know the numbers. There is a formula I'm going to give you here that you will be using to calculate your starting point in calories for each day and how many calories you can eat each day in order to lose a certain number of pounds per week. Yes it will be that simple! As I said before, the hard part is the tracking.

Now, there are many of these formulas floating around out there. I have found them all almost identical in the numbers they produce. I believe mine came from *Men's Health* magazine, and I found another good one from the *American Heart Association*, but stick with mine and you'll do great I promise. Here it is.

- Take your current weight and write it down.

- Multiply that number by 11.

- Now, if you don't exercise at all, add 20% *of* that number **to** that number.

- If you feel you get moderate exercise, add 30% instead of 20%.

- If you're an exercise maniac (4–6 days per week), then add 40% instead of 20%

This number you're now looking at is the exact number of calories you can eat in any given day and stay exactly the same weight you started the day at. Here's an example using the exact numbers I started with when I began this Stage:

My Weight = 220 lbs.
220 X 11 = 2420.
2420 X 20% = 484
2420 + 484 = 2904.

My number started out at 2904. This was the number of calories I could eat every day and not lose or gain a pound. It sounds like a lot, and it should! Even at 220 lbs., I was a big person! Not like I was at 268, but still very large. The bigger you are and the more you weigh, the higher this starting number is going to be. The higher the starting number, the easier it will seem to others for you to be able to handle because you can have more calories per day.

I will say that for those of you starting at 150 pounds and have a starting number of 1980 calories, you will think you've got it a lot tougher than the rest, but

I'm telling you that this is not so! You didn't consume nearly the quantity of food before that the others did. Everything is relative. It will be just as hard for them to cut down calories as it will be for you.

Now let's check out the last part of the formula. For every 500 calories you cut from that _**daily**_ number you just finished calculating, you will lose 1 pound per _**week.**_

So, looking at my example above. If I had kept my calorie intake at 2404 per day, I would have lost 1 pound per week. 1904 calories per day would have equated to 2 pounds per week, and so on. ***THIS IS ABSOLUTELY, POSITIVELY, 100% ACCURATE AND FOOLPROOF AND WILL WORK EVERY TIME NO MATTER WHAT YOUR STARTING WEIGHT.***

Now, I'm going to let that sink in for a bit and talk a little about exercise at this point, before I go into the details about how to calculate your daily calorie intake to the exactness required for success. Just start thinking about your number, and don't worry yet how low it may seem to you. You will see that you can make this work!

The Exercise Factor

Up until now, I've said that exercise was not necessary for my plan. Don't worry! I haven't changed that! I would, however, be foolish if I didn't tell you that exercise is very beneficial to you for many reasons, including, but not limited to, the following:

- You will lose weight quicker.

- You will get rid of excess fat and flab sooner.

- You will create a more toned look for your new body.

- You will feel much better every day and have much more energy than before.

You'll notice that I used the 20% calculation in my formula for figuring out my starting calorie number earlier. I was exercising daily, and probably could have used the 30% or 40% addition, but I chose not to, and would advise you to do the same. I say just use the 20% figure in your calculation no matter what, then any exercise you do is gravy (so to speak) and will show in your weekly weight loss number.

I felt, and still feel, that if I allowed myself more calories each day, then I would feel more obligated to exercise in order to counteract them. Obligation creates more stress! Since the only variable in the formula that's not exact is the exercise factor, I just use the lowest number and get better results the more I exercise.

Now I will never tell you to go join a gym, or buy equipment of any kind for your house. If you want to do those things, it's totally up to you. I did not. All I did was start getting some cardiovascular exercise around the house and with the kids in order to get about 20 minutes to an hour per day of exercise.

I have 2 young children. When I started Stage 4, I had 1 child, Parker, who was going on 2 years old. As soon as the weather warmed up (I had started Stage 4 in winter), I started putting Parker in the baby seat attached to my bicycle and riding around my neighborhood for about 20–30 minutes each night after dinner. By the end of that summer, it had turned into an hour each night!

I was feeling stronger and healthier than ever with great amounts of energy compared to my former self. I hadn't exercised regularly in prior years, so I worked my way up gradually, but with the bike riding, it didn't take long.

Also at the end of the summer, I made the best $150 purchase I have ever made in my life. I bought a portable basketball hoop for my driveway, the kind that has a base you fill with water and is adjustable from 8–10 feet. I put Parker's baby basketball hoop next to it, and we started playing in the driveway every night thereafter.

Then, when winter came again, I had nothing but an exercise bike in the house, and I did use it for a few weeks at the start of the season, but I'm here to tell you that I stopped soon thereafter, didn't use it again for the rest of the winter, and still lost my 2–3 pounds every week I was on my plan.

So I got rid of the exercise bike, and I'll say again, the exercise is not necessary. You *will* lose the weight if you follow the calorie counting method. PERIOD!

The next spring, I brought the basketball hoop out of the shed, and started playing every night with my son, and that's all I have been doing since, even to this day. Since we had our second child, Evan, in May that year, I couldn't do the bike rides anymore, since Evan wasn't big enough for the seat. I could, however, have him outside with me in a stroller or a contained area while Parker and I played basketball.

Today I weigh about 190 lbs., look more toned then I ever did back in high school when I used to work out and play sports (or try to!) regularly, and all I do is play 20 minutes to an hour of basketball in my driveway each and every night.

The reason I look better now than I did back then is because my exercise is combined with **much** healthier eating. Back in my younger days, I sure didn't eat any vegetables!

I only skip a night when it rains or when I have some other obligation of course. I take care of my 2 young children each night, as my wife works most nights at the hospital, so those of you who think you don't have time to do this, I don't know what to say to you.

Again, it's not required, but it will help you get to where you want to be much quicker and help you get healthy and stay healthy for the rest of your life!

THE LOGIC BEHIND STAGE 4

The logic here should seem easy, since it's based on science this time. If you keep the calories exactly where you should according to the formula, you will lose the specified weight each week until you reach your goal.

The logic for your mind, and the way I saw this at the time, is to understand just where you've been and what you've been doing up to this point. You see, technically, you've been cutting calories ever since Stage 1! You just didn't term it this way and you didn't have to do any math or put together any spreadsheets. That's why I believe my plan is so unique and wonderful!

Before you started my plan, you were eating tremendous amounts of junk all day, every day. When you did eat regular meals, they were very high in fat, cholesterol, and of course, calories. You were a very large, overweight person because of all the calories you were eating.

I've read that it takes 3500 calories to gain 1 pound. To most people, 3500 calories sounds impossible to reach! You wouldn't believe it, but the thin people out there wouldn't know *how* to eat that much in a day!

We know better. We used to eat that amount of calories as an appetizer before breakfast! Seriously, you weren't adding them up before because you didn't care. I'm telling you in all seriousness that you and I were eating more like 35,000 calories in a day than 3500, and that's why we were 50 pounds or more (some a lot more) overweight.

So in Stage 1, you cut calories by changing not how much you were eating, but **what** you were eating, and the new foods were much lower in fat **and calories** than the foods you were eating before, so you lost weight per the formula you didn't even know about yet.

In Stage 2, you stopped eating late, and therefore cut back in calories just because you took away a portion of the day you were allowed to eat during! You still may have felt you ate just as much in Stage 2 as you did in Stage 1, but I'm here to tell you that you didn't! It wasn't possible you see. There just was less time each day for you to stuff your face, so therefore, you consumed fewer calories!

The added benefit to Stage 2 was twofold. You stopped putting calories into your body late at night that couldn't be burned off, *and* you prepped your mind to be ready for the rest of your life, when eating junk at night will not be amenable to maintaining a healthy, great-looking body!

In Stage 3 you cut portions, therefore you cut calories. It was as simple as that! You also stopped eating as much sugar, which turns into calories, and salt, which retains water weight.

So now, in Stage 4, you're finally at the place where you will be looking in detail at the calories you're eating in order to cut them back to a level where you can lose more weight!

For those of you just looking to lose those vanity pounds and starting at Stage 4, it's the same principle for you, just not to the scale. You're a nibbler. You didn't think you were eating too many calories, but since you weren't keeping track, a little bit here and a little bit there added up to too many.

If you don't regulate the amount of calories you're eating and keep track of it, you will not be able to lose those extra pounds and keep them off. Sure you can just cut back on food altogether and lose the weight, but it always comes back, and that's why you're reading this book!

By now, you should understand why I called my plan The Logic Diet. It should all make just as much sense to you now as it did to me when I was coming up with it.

Now, are you ready to start counting calories? For those of you with me the whole way, make sure you always follow the rules set forth in **all** of the prior Stages as you work through Stage 4.

THE IMPORTANCE OF SERVING SIZE

So you know exactly how many calories you can eat every day in order to lose 2 or 3 pounds per week, but how do you really measure what you're putting into your mouth? Well that answer is strict. You need to know *exactly* how many calories that *every single thing* you eat has in it.

If this is the case, then to start with, you need to know *exactly how much* of that thing you're actually eating. What I mean by this is that you have to *exactly measure your serving sizes.*

Now this may sound more complicated than it is, but it's about the most important thing to learn, so you must get it right. On every nutritional label on any product out there that has one, there is a measure of serving size and servings per container, or something similar, listed on the packaging.

If what you're eating is 1 slice of fat free cheese, and the package lists the serving size as 1 slice, then you know exactly how many calories are in that slice of cheese. If what you're eating is ½ of a *brick* of fat free cheese, and the serving size is ¼ brick, then you need to double the number of calories, since it's listed as *calories per serving*. Make sense? It needs to, so we'll keep on it.

Many of them get more complicated, so you might even need your calculator handy! For example, if what you're eating lists the serving size in ounces or grams or cups, etc., you'll probably need to use the servings per container number to figure it out.

Say you're having ½ bag of frozen vegetables, and it says the serving size is 1 cup. Well, that really helps (not)! So you have to look at the servings per bag, and it says "around 5." Let's say it tells you that there are 30 calories per serving. You figure this by equating ½ bag to 2½ servings. Then multiply 30 times 2½ to get 75 calories.

You are going to have to do this with absolutely everything you are eating, all day long, so you can have the exact number of calories to plug into the formula. You will soon know just which foods you can keep on your plan and which ones have to go because you can't afford the calories. You'll be able to plan out your meals and keep the total calories for your day under the limit you need to achieve your weekly weight loss goal.

Does this sound like too much work? Well first I'll say **TOO BAD!** You'll thank me for it later! Next I'll say that if you start a chart when you do this, or even just scratch it down on paper whenever you figure out how much of a certain food you eat when you eat it and the corresponding calories *for that serving* *size*, then you'll never have to do it for that particular food again (as long as you always eat the same serving size each time, which you probably will)!

You might think that the list will get too long, but if you're having to stay below 2000 calories per day or even lower (some of you much lower), you'll find that, before too long, your list of foods you eat, with the portions you eat and the calories for that portion listed, will be complete.

Then all you'll need is your list and you'll be able to do the math every day just by looking at it and choosing items from your own personal "menu" to eat for your 3 meals that day. You'll be able to add things to this "menu" whenever you want as long as it meets all the qualifications of the prior Stages and allows you to stay under your calorie goal each day. Remember, you still must eat 3 meals each day!

Once you practice judging how much you eat of each food and how your serving size equates to the calories listed on the package, you'll become an expert in no time, and it'll really open your eyes as to just how many calories are in food! You won't believe it sometimes. You'll certainly better understand why more people out there are overweight!

DON'T LEAVE ANYTHING OUT

You're figuring out how to measure and calculate calories for what you're eating, but make sure you don't forget the first thing I said in the last section. That is to measure the calories in ***every single thing*** you're eating.

When I started Stage 4, I questioned whether I would have to figure out the calories for vegetables since they were usually freebies on other diet plans, but I needed my formula to be accurate, so I set out to figure them out.

Since they usually have no labels (some do if you're lucky enough), I had to go on the internet to find out. What I found, thank goodness, was a lot of sites that had the information I was seeking. All you have to do is go to a search engine and do a web search for "calorie counters."

You'll find many places to look up anything from an egg to a cucumber or anything else you can think of and get the calories per serving you need to fill in the blanks. Some of them even list the information in the same nutritional label format you'd see at the market! Again, my favorite is free and is at www.nutritiondata.com.

The other thing I was leaving out until I caught myself, and I'll bet you'd do it too if I didn't say anything, are the **condiments** you're using. That's right! Ketchup has calories. A1 Steak Sauce has calories. Fat free mayonnaise has calories. Get the point? You absolutely must look at those labels as well and add those calories into your equation.

Yes, you have to figure out your serving size as well! I try to figure it out in tablespoons using a guess as close as I can get. Most condiments have their measurements listed in tablespoons. If you do it that way, you'll most likely only be a couple calories off if you're guessing, and that won't hurt any.

What *would* hurt is if you left the condiments out altogether. They could be the difference between losing 1 or 2 pounds per week, and could seriously hurt your mental state if you couldn't figure out why the weight loss isn't what you thought it'd be each week.

What I did to help this is to actually figure the condiments right into my menu listings, including the portion of the condiment I use with the portion of the food I use it with. For example, on my list would be "1 lean burger patty with A1 Steak sauce = 260 calories." I would have checked out the portion size of the sauce I used and just calculated it into the whole meal item.

PLANNING THE DAY

Now that you've done your homework, made your listings, and figured out the calories of everything you're eating (you'll be adding things to the list all the time), you should make a plan for your day at first, just until you get used to monitoring your calories like this.

I mean it's tough to stay below a number if you hit it by lunchtime. You need structure until you can wing it and still stay within the calorie range you need to be in.

To do this the right way, in my opinion, is to separate it out into the 3 meals, then figure out the foods you are going to eat during each meal in advance, add up the calories, then make sure you add or subtract in order to stay at the level you need.

You'll notice I said *add* here. That's right! I do not intend for you to go under the calories you need to lose, say, 2 pounds per week, just because you think it'll be easier to starve yourself and lose weight quicker.

I want you to decide whether you want to lose 1, 2, 3, or 4 pounds per week at this Stage (NO MORE THAN 4 IS ACCEPTABLE, AND I BET YOUR DOCTOR WOULD TELL YOU THE SAME!), then make sure you eat right up to the calorie number you need in order to lose at that level. If the formula says you can eat 1500 calories to lose 2 pounds per week, *THEN EAT 1500 CALORIES!* Not less!

Here is an example of a plan, complete with accurate food listings, which I would use to get me through a typical day.

BREAKFAST:

- 2 slices of fat free toast (70 calories) with unlimited spray butter (0 calories) and 4 tablespoons total of sugar free jelly (40 calories) = 110 calories.

- My berry mixture which includes 3 tablespoons sugar free Cool Whip (45 calories), ½ package frozen mixed berries (88 calories), and 1 container of Dannon Light 'N Fit Yogurt (60 calories) = 193 calories

- 2 cups of coffee with 2 tablespoons fat free creamer and unlimited sugar substitute (0 calories) = 66 calories

TOTAL BREAKFAST CALORIES = 369

LUNCH:

- **_2_** sandwiches, each containing 2 slices of fat free bread (70 calories), 1 slice of fat free cheese (30 calories), 2 slices of fat free bologna (40 calories), and unlimited mustard (0 calories) = 280 calories

- 1 container of the yogurt = 60 calories

- 1 container of sugar free Jello = 10 calories

- Diet pop or bottled water = 0 calories

- 1 banana (about 8") = 100 calories

TOTAL LUNCH CALORIES = 450

DINNER:

- 2 lean burger patties (340 calories) with 4 tablespoons A1 steak sauce (90 calories) = 430 calories

- 1 package frozen broccoli and cauliflower mixed vegetables with unlimited spray butter = 125 calories

- 1 large baked potato with unlimited spray butter = 100 calories

- 1 salad made from 4 cups of lettuce (24 calories), ½ tomato (diced) (11 calories), ½ cup sliced cucumber (7 calories), and unlimited calorie free salad dressing = 42 calories

- Diet pop or bottled water = 0 calories

TOTAL DINNER CALORIES = 697

TOTAL CALORIES FOR THE DAY = 1516

Most of you are probably thinking that this seems like quite a lot of food in the day for only 1516 calories, and you're right! You're not starving yourself on this plan! This just goes to show you just how much of a difference the low-fat and fat-free foods truly make in your calorie intake, and why Stages 1 and 2 were so successful for you.

Here is another example for those of you who need even fewer calories. I'm using most of the same foods here, but you can be substituting anything you're using from your own personal menu items of course.

BREAKFAST:

- Coffee (as before) = 66 calories

- My berry mixture (as before) = 193 calories

- 2 slices of fat free toast with unlimited spray butter and NO jelly = 70 calories

TOTAL BREAKFAST CALORIES = 329

LUNCH:

- 1 fat free bologna and cheese sandwich (as before) = 140 calories

- 1 container of yogurt (as before) = 60 calories

- 1 container of sugar free pudding = 60 calories

- Diet pop or water = 0 calories

TOTAL LUNCH CALORIES = 260

DINNER:

- 1 salad (as before) = 42 calories

- 1 package mixed frozen vegetables (as before) = 125 calories

- 1 lean burger patty (170 calories) and 2 tablespoons A1 steak sauce (45 calories) = 215 calories

- 1 baked potato with unlimited spray butter = 100 calories

TOTAL DINNER CALORIES = 482

TOTAL CALORIES FOR THE DAY = 1071

These are just examples! You will be using all different kinds of foods that you came to love during the first 3 Stages of this plan and mixing it up in the ways that you like best.

You'll see now why I said earlier that you'd have to eliminate some of the other foods that were OK during Stage 1 and 2. You just don't have the calorie allowance for some of them, especially those with sugar in them.

I don't even eat bananas anymore, since I like to replace those calories with more, lower calorie things now, but you can get a grasp on how this will work for you. If you like dessert, and want to have a pint of strawberries (only 114 calories) after dinner and skip the baked potato, then go ahead! A large sweet potato (which has about 162 calories) is also a great substitute for a regular baked potato during dinner and almost feels like a special treat.

Speaking of dinner, you'll see in the example how I still save my biggest meal with the most calories for last. I still have to get through the rest of the night, and have always had success doing it that way.

For those of you who think you can't eat a lot of food in Stage 4, try those dinners listed above. Some of you won't even be able to finish all of that! It's good old-fashioned meat, potatoes, vegetables, and salad!

You can see how this will be an exact science. If you follow this to the letter, you will reap the benefits exactly as described by the formula. Once you master it, you'll be able to tweak it any way you want to.

You can even end up going to the fast food restaurants' web sites, download their menus and calorie listings, and incorporate the low fat, low calorie items into your plan. I don't recommend doing this until Stage 5, but I'm just showing you how this will change your life forever.

You'll always be able to use the tactics and information in this section in order to monitor yourself, and it will be a big help to you in maintaining your body once you get to your goal weight.

CHEATING ON STAGE 4

So, you've got your list, you're working hard every day to stay right at your limit of calories, and you're seeing the results. You've been on it for 3 weeks, let's say, and have already lost 10 pounds! The first week that you're on Stage 4, you should see faster results because you're going to lose a little water weight, and you're really monitoring calories for the first time to this level.

Now, depending on how long it's been since you've done any cheat days (or half days), you may be getting a little edgy. No matter how gradually you're led through this process and up to this Stage, I never said it would be easy! You're doing something you've probably never done before, and your mind and body are going to have to get used to it.

This is where I have my best news for you! When it comes to cheating on this Stage, believe it or not, the rules are not going to change from the previous Stages!

You heard me right! When you cheat here, you can do the same cheating you've always done on this plan. You can eat whatever you want for a day, or a half-day, not caring when or what it is you're eating. As I've said before, if you're going to cheat, cheat RIGHT!

Make sure you reward yourself for the hardship you're putting yourself through. The part you're probably going to find a little amusing once you're to this point however, is that you're not going to find these cheat days as rewarding now as they were a few months ago. You may not even eat as much as you did before, since your stomach is smaller now and you can't eat as much anyway.

You may even be really surprised with yourself because you find you don't even crave some of the same foods you used to anymore! You have changed your entire life and the way you nourish your body, and your mind has dramatically changed as well.

Now for the rest of you (as is the case with me), there will be some foods you will ALWAYS crave. So on your cheat days have as much of those as you want!

Just remember the basic rules of cheating I gave you in Stage 2 as regards the math involved. It will still work the same now. 1 day off will take 3 days on to get back to the prior weight. It will still hold true every time!

We will only start messing with the rules of cheating when you're in Stage 5, so you still have a lot of time to truly enjoy those cheat days. As you go longer and longer on Stage 4, you'll find yourself not wanting to cheat as often. You'll find yourself getting closer and closer to your weight loss goals, and you'll be able to project out just when you should get there. Therefore, your mind will stop you from taking those cheat days.

You'll be amazed, but you'll have a chance to cheat, or you'll have an occasion to cheat, and you won't! Once you get to this level and your mind is doing these sorts of things, you should really congratulate yourself. This means you're pretty much at the mental state you'll need to attain to be able to keep this weight off forever.

It means your brain has been conditioned more to being a thin person than a fat person. That transition will become more complete over the next few Stages, but it's a great accomplishment at this point.

This is the main reason why most other diet plans won't help you forever. It's because your mind can't make that complete transition into **believing** you're a thin person now. This plan accomplishes that for you.

THE END OF STAGE 4 (A MONUMENTAL OCCASION!)

The end of this Stage is truly a thing to behold. It comes a lot quicker than you thought it would. If you've been with me from the beginning, it could be anywhere from 6 months to a year before you're here, but it still seems like it's been fast.

You have been clicking along on the plan, losing 2–3 pounds per week, then taking some cheat days or a vacation, coming back, picking up where you left off, etc…for so long now it's become your life's routine. You no longer have the stress involved with losing weight. It's natural for you now.

Others envy you and compliment you on a daily basis. If you're married, your spouse has taken a *whole* new interest in your body that I'm sure you've been very pleased with. You may have even noticed your spouse changing him or herself a little trying to keep up with you.

This is because you spouse is now becoming a little (or a lot) worried! That's right! If you notice that you're being treated a lot nicer than you used to be, it's because your spouse is worried you may leave him or her for someone else now that you look so thin and sexy. It's also because they notice the way the opposite sex has been looking at you lately!

Take advantage of this as much as you can, because it won't last for a long time. Once your spouse gets used to your new look, things will go right back to the way they used to be.

If you're single, then you've already been taking advantage of the results you've been getting I'm sure! It's unfortunate that the social standards in this country are the way they are, but at least now you're rolling with it! You're thinner, sexier, and are getting a whole lot more attention than you're used to getting from the opposite sex.

I'd say at this point, you need to get with some of your friends that have always been thinner and sexier for some pointers on how to use this new look of yours to your advantage.

Anyway, if you're here, then you've hit your goal! You have lost all the weight you wanted to lose, and the scale is now your friend every morning. You may have been like me and lowered your final goal several times before you ended up here since it was so easy to do so.

You found out using my foolproof method, adjusted to the fat free foods you picked for yourself to eat on a regular basis, that after a while you could monitor your calories each day without putting much thought into it, and lose weight every week on schedule.

You need to celebrate! You've made it! Way to go! Congratulations!

The one thing I would say is to NOT celebrate with a cheat day! You want to prove to yourself that you don't need bad foods in order to enjoy yourself. You are getting ready to set up Stages 5 and 6, which are the maintenance phases that you will be employing for the rest of your life, in order to stave off the critics and negative people you've been dealing with who've said you'd never make it and keep the weight off.

Celebrate by going out with your friends or with your spouse for a night out dancing or whatever it may be as long as it doesn't involve food. You're going to need to condition your mind to not associate food with reward anymore. I know I've let you cheat in full on all Stages of this plan, but from now on, you're going to have to tail off of that.

The logic behind this was that, during the first 4 Stages, you were conditioning yourself to change your life. You needed as much mental support to do this as possible. Letting you have great cheat rewards helped you cope with the complete change you were going through.

Now that you've completed the change, the only thing left to do is maintain what you've worked so hard to accomplish. I'm going to, of course, help you through this as well, and I believe it is the hardest thing to do.

It's much harder than actually losing the weight, and that's because your mind tells you that you're now done! You've made it! You don't have to diet anymore!

Well, that's kind of right and it's kind of wrong. You don't have to diet to *lose* weight anymore, but you still have to "diet" to maintain your weight so you don't ruin all that long and hard work.

As I said, the end came along faster than you would have thought, and so you're saying to yourself "What do I do now?" "How do I go forward with this from now on?" Without a plan for this, your brain would just go crazy and you'd slip back to old habits. You have to be more careful now than ever before to make sure you don't revert to your old ways.

Like a life-long smoker, it wouldn't take much to get back on that bad food wagon and, next thing you know, start to get heavier again. If that happens, your mind doesn't want to go through the work of losing the weight back, and you're in a vicious cycle.

I don't mean to scare you! I just want to be sure you fully understand that the work is not over. Congratulations on getting to your goal! You deserve a lot of credit. I'm glad I could help you get here. If you stay with me, I will help you make sure you ***never*** go back!

ANOTHER LOOK AT PLATEAUS

As I stated during Stage 1, a plateau is where you are stuck at a certain weight for at least a few days, usually about a week, but not more than 2 weeks. Once you are stuck for 2 weeks, you move on to the next level of weight loss.

At this point, your plateau should be at your goal weight of course! If you still have more weight to lose on Stage 4, and your plateau has lasted more than 2 weeks, then you simply are not counting calories correctly or are not using the formula correctly. I say again here that it is 100% accurate and foolproof if followed correctly.

Don't second guess yourself, or start to question the validity of the formula and that it works. This is easy to do since you're on unfamiliar ground and you mind is new to this way of thinking.

There are also texts and articles floating around out there that say something to the effect that they believe your body adjusts to your calorie intake drop and starts to burn the exact amount of calories you are now eating. For instance, they'll say that if you start eating 1000 calories per day, your body will start burning only 1000 calories per day and therefore you stop losing weight, and this is what's causing your plateau.

This is such utter hogwash that I can't believe anyone would fall for it. They are saying this in order to sell you (for at least $25 and sometimes a lot more) on whatever their plan may be that is, of course, against calorie counting. If what they say were true, there would be no such thing as anorexia in the world. People could just stop eating altogether and just stay at the same weight because their bodies would just stop burning calories!

Sounds amazingly idiotic, doesn't it? That's because it is. Now remember, I'm not a doctor and I'm not schooled in the exact science of these things, but the formula I presented in Stage 4 of this plan works because everyone's body burns calories based on their size. That's why your doctor has a chart where they can look up what your ideal weight should be based upon your height. They call this the body mass index or BMI.

I'm 6'2". According to the BMI, I would be considered overweight if I weighed between 194 and 232 pounds. I would be considered obese if I weighed 233 pounds or higher. Remember I started this plan at 268 pounds! I was definitely obese! I am now maintaining at about 190 pounds. Now I'm not even considered overweight at all!

Now sure, everyone is different. These are averages and some people are lucky and have a much faster metabolism and some people are unlucky and have biological conditions that cause their metabolisms to be much slower. However, most are very close to the average and that's why calorie counting is successful.

Some of you who have slightly slower metabolisms will find the plan takes a little longer because you've only lost 1–2 pounds per week instead of 3–4, but the fact is that the plan still worked! Those of you with biological conditions causing extremely slow metabolism should be working with your doctor for treatment and a specific weight loss plan based on your individual needs. Those with faster metabolisms aren't reading this because they're the ones who don't have to diet at all!

Now as your weight drops, it takes fewer calories to maintain that weight, so you must take in fewer and fewer calories in order to lose weight. The rate at which your body is burning those calories is the constant! It's not going to change! This is why the formula works! This is also why so many fad diet pills out there claim to boost your metabolism so you can lose more weight without eating fewer calories. These are more things trying to separate you from your hard-earned money.

So why are you having the plateau then? Well it's simply because your body is continually adjusting to the changes you're making in your diet and calorie intake. Your body is designed to protect itself from death. When you drop weight as significantly as you're doing it, the body, from time to time, must make sure that it's not going to starve to death.

So, in my humble opinion, the body ***temporarily*** stops burning the calories necessary to lose weight in order to perform a sort of self-test to be sure that the operating system (you) isn't going to kill it! So for at least 3 and as many as 10 days, you stay at the same weight until the body adjusts to the amount of calories you're taking in, then slowly raises its metabolism back to level where the calories will be burned.

Since you are then keeping your calorie intake at or about the same level, the body continues to burn calories at its normal rate and you're back to losing 3–4 pounds per week again. You typically won't have another plateau for at least a month, but as you get thinner and lose more weight, the plateaus come more often. When you were really heavy, you didn't really have any of them!

Let's face it; the end of Stage 1 wasn't a plateau, you just stopped losing because you needed to decrease calories some more. When you got to Stage 4, you had more plateaus because it's the first time your body may have felt it was in danger!

The plateaus are also why I recommended that you eat right up to the allowable calories per day in order to lose about up to 4 pounds per week but no more.

If you tried to lose weight too fast, aside from being very unhealthy, you would have many more plateaus since the body would see the faster weight loss as even more of a threat, and wouldn't get used to a consistent calorie intake level in order to get off of that plateau faster!

I hope this helped to allay your fears about the plateaus you've had or are having, and helped you to understand why they occur. If you stick to the plan and the formula, and make sure you're doing it absolutely correctly, then you will have no problems. Most of you are not having the problems, so this has just helped to boost your confidence even higher going into the maintenance Stages!

Review Before Moving Forward

At this point, I think it's prudent to take a look back at the journey you've taken thus far in order to look ahead at what you need to do next.

Once I got to my goal weight, I was almost at a loss as to what to do next. You see, I never really thought I would make it to my final goal. I was making this up as I went along, and I guess part of me wasn't totally sure it would really work. I knew what I was doing was logical, and that it was healthy, and that my weight was dropping as it should, but I still was shocked when I reached my final goal of 190 pounds!

I had lost 78 pounds, and was as thin as I was over 15 years earlier when I was still in college. I knew that if I continued to follow the principles I had set for myself up to this point, I would never gain the weight back, but I hadn't really prepared yet for the maintenance phase of the plan. I was so focused on getting there that I hadn't thought out what to do once I got there.

I have figured that out since and will relay that to you in Stages 5 and 6, but now we'll look at the steps we've been following. You will still need to follow most of these principles for the rest of your days if you want to keep the weight off, so it's worth the time to review.

At this point, we're doing the following on a daily basis:

1. Eating low-fat (or non-fat) and low-calorie foods, usually staying below 25 grams of fat per day.

2. Weighing yourself every day, at the same time.

3. Eating 3 meals each and every day.

4. Taking a daily multivitamin and a calcium supplement.

5. Not eating after 7:00 PM (or later than 4 hours prior to bedtime)

6. Not using extra salt or sugar, and eating low-sugar foods or foods using sugar substitutes.

7. Monitoring the exact calories in everything you eat.

8. Calculating the exact amount of calories you eat at each meal and using the total for the day in your weight loss formula to determine how many pounds per week you'll lose.

9. Taking full cheat days or half-days off of the diet as a reward.

10. Going off of the plan completely during vacations, holidays, or special occasions.

11. Maybe you're exercising regularly, and maybe you're not.

Does that about sum it up? Does it look easy now? Can you believe that you've really been doing this all this time now? It almost all seems too easy when you look at it like this doesn't it? Very funny right!

Again, most of these things you will continue to do in one form or another for the rest of your life. You are not going to be able to just stop doing these things or you WILL gain all of the weight back.

As I've said many times, I've led you to this point extremely gradually over many months in order to convert your mind into the mind of a thinner person. This is why you've succeeded up to this point, and it's why you WILL succeed from now on!

So revel in the fact that you've hit your goal! Brag to everyone that you are now finished with the weight loss part of your life!

Next we'll discuss in Stage 5 how to keep yourself where you are now, and in Stage 6, we'll get into having a little more fun with what you're eating.

Stage 5

Maintaining Your New Body

Step back. Look in the mirror. Get on the scale. That's right, you did it! I know you still don't believe it, but you did it! So now what?! How the heck are you going to keep this weight off? You're now an expert in losing the weight, and your mind is conditioned for the rigors of that task, but now you have to switch gears into maintenance mode. I'm here to tell you that this is, in my opinion, the hardest part of the whole process.

I say that because now you don't have a goal anymore. There's nothing to shoot for. There's no motivation to forge ahead day after day trying to attain a certain end that's always in the front of your mind. It's almost anticlimactic. However, you must now make sure your mental state is as strong as ever, because you must make sure you never slip back into any of your former patterns of thought when it comes to food.

Whatever you do, you must not allow yourself to feel you can now celebrate your achievement by eating whatever you want again! DO NOT take a cheat day right after you hit your goal weight! You need to continue on right into this Stage so that your mind will get used to the idea of keeping yourself steady at the new weight and body you've created.

Actually, you will have a goal again, it's just more of an abstract goal than a concrete one. It's more of an idea. The goal is to keep your weight at no more than 5 pounds lighter or heavier than your goal weight at all times. In order to accomplish this, you are going to have to continue to monitor what you eat every single day. It will be just as tasking, if not more, than it was on Stage 4 because you have to be just as vigilant in keeping this weight off as you were losing it in the first place.

It's lucky for you that the logic behind this is just as easy to grasp. It will make sense to you, and it will follow in the context of everything you have learned so far.

A New Goal Means New Math

The path to maintenance is to continue the rigorous monitoring of Stage 4, just in a new way in order to stay put instead of losing more weight. Do not fall into the trap of thinking you might as well just keep lowering your goal weight and continue to lose more and more weight. Your goal was not to become anorexic, just to get healthy and get to your goal weight.

If you think you should lose more just because you can, I suggest you contact your doctor and let him or her advise you on the healthiest weight for your size and body type.

OK, do you remember the math we used in Stage 4? All you have to do is start the formula again and find out what your daily maximum calorie intake is right now. Then, instead of subtracting from that number in order to lose a certain number of pounds per week, you'll just try to *hit* that number so you don't gain or lose any weight.

In my case, my final weight was 190 pounds. 190 X 11 = 2090. 2090 X 20% = 418. 2090 + 418 = 2508. That was it! If I ate 2508 calories per day (or right around there), I was going to stay right where I was. Again, this is FOOLPROOF AND WILL WORK EVERY TIME FOR EVERYBODY!

Now, I know what you're thinking. You're saying "I don't want to have to count calories every single day for the rest of my life!" I agree with you and I promise you won't have to do that. However, at the *start* of your maintenance phase, you will **NEED** to do this. You are not ready to just start changing your very structured life that you created in order to get where you are now into an *unstructured* way of eating.

You will need to *gradually* lead yourself off of the calorie counting just like you *gradually* led your mind through the weight-loss process.

I don't need to tell you in detail at this point how to get your calorie intake to where it needs to be. You are an expert by now at adding and deleting foods from your daily diet as necessary in order to be at a certain number of calories per day. All you have to do is add to your foods each day in order to hit the new number.

Now don't add any non-approved foods! You still must stick to ALL of the rules from ALL of the prior Stages. This includes staying on the supplements I recommended.

Soon enough you'll be changing up the foods you eat again, but for now stick to what's been successful for you to this point. You'll need to transition very slowly into Stage 6, which is where you'll start adding other foods back into your diet.

THE LOGIC BEHIND STAGE 5

You'll notice that when I used my example above of how many calories I was going to eat during each day to maintain my new weight, I used the 20% addition again. I exercise now much more than I did even during Stages 3 and 4, but as before, I just allow that to count as extra for me instead of bumping my eating knowing I'll "work it off" later.

This works great in Stage 5 as well. You can add the extra calories, then exercise helps you stay at the weight even easier, while also helping you tone up that new body of yours. For those of you not exercising, the formula still works great!

The logic behind this Stage is that you still keep your **mind** structured when you start your maintenance.

If you try to go off the plan cold turkey (so to speak), you'll most likely not be able to control yourself, and then you'll start to consume too many calories and fat grams. Then you'll find yourself back on Stage 4 trying to lose the weight all over again.

You need to get to where you're not just gaining every week and then losing it back the next. This is what happened to me at first as I tried to figure out what I was going to do after Stage 4 and before I figured out that I needed to keep the heavy structure and the calorie counting going.

Before I learned that very important point, I was taking a few days off completely each week, then using Stage 4 methodology to lose the weight back the following week. I thought I could use this as a maintenance plan forever, but I was *extremely* wrong.

It's very important that you remind yourself of one of the things you learned in Stage 1. You will have to give up foods you love. Just amend it a little bit at this point and say the following: You will have to give up the foods you love *in the manner that you used to eat them.*

Does this make sense? Hopefully it will become clearer as we progress through Stage 6. In a nutshell, it's not like you'll never eat pizza again. You just might end up having a slice or two instead of a whole 16-inch pie by yourself.

It's not like you'll never eat at McDonald's again. You just might end up having 1 double cheeseburger and a side salad instead of 3 double cheeseburgers and fries. It's not like you'll never have cake again. You just might end up having one medium size piece instead of 2 large pieces and everyone else's leftovers.

Have you noticed how most people leave a quarter to a half of their piece of cake uneaten? It's amazing isn't it?

This whole change is a major thing for you, but it's a regular way of life for thin people. When you see thin people eat the foods you used to eat a ton of, you can't believe they can stay thin while eating them.

However, they have never eaten them in the sheer *quantities* that you used to. They have always eaten in **moderation**. Wow! There's that word for the first time. **MODERATION**. What a concept! This is the logic behind your new life. This should be your call signal. This should be your battle cry! Keep this word in your mind at all times for the rest of your days.

Hopefully, soon enough, this will become second nature to you just like it is with all of the other thin people you've seen out there. Hopefully, it will become instinctual. It will take a lot of time! Don't think that just because it took you a long time to lose the weight that the time served is over!

It's going to take, in my opinion, *years* in order to totally convert yourself into a thin person with a thin person's mentality. Don't let this discourage you! It should motivate you! You can do this! Look what you've accomplished thus far.

You have the knowledge going for you that, even if it takes a long time to become instinctual for you, you have Stage 4 of my plan to fall back on. To this day, if I find myself gaining a few pounds because my internal moderation monitoring system was malfunctioning a bit, I just go right back on Stage 4 until I'm back at my goal weight, which usually only takes 3–5 days.

By this point, Stage 4 should be like a comfort zone for you. It's something you're very at ease with. You'll feel safe when you're on it, since you know the success of it is 100% guaranteed.

MODERATION TAKES BABY STEPS

This whole thing may sound troubling to you. I told you that I believe this to be the hardest step in the process of changing your life and mental state! I still have to work at this every single day in order to keep my body where I want it to be.

I have been on my maintenance phase for over a year and still have to monitor myself quite a bit. Every time I see my reflection in something, or see myself in a picture or on a home movie, I'm reminded of why it's all worthwhile.

Look at yourself! Keep reminding yourself of how great you look! Your body will start to become more toned and muscular looking as well as thinner. Every time you get a second (or third) glance from the opposite sex, you should feel much better at how much work this is for you!

OK. Step away from the mirror for a second and let's get back to how to take those steps toward moderation and not having to count calories every single day.

Whether or not you have to monitor those calories daily, you definitely should ***not stop*** weighing yourself every day. No matter what I've read out there, I still say you need to weigh yourself daily, and at the same time daily, in order to have a firm grasp on what you need to be doing that day or that week in order to keep your weight under control.

I don't care whether you've been at your goal weight for a couple years or a couple months. I still weigh myself every day, and I will continue to do so, probably forever. It's always a good thing to remind yourself where it is you've come from, and how hard it was for you to get here. You've silenced all your critics. You've shown everyone you could do it. So keep track of what you're doing every day so you don't throw it all away.

So how do you go back to eating certain foods in moderation while keeping your calorie intake where it needs to be so you don't gain too much weight back? You have to take baby steps in order to do this and keep your mind converting itself at the right pace.

The first baby step you will take is just adding to Stage 4 until you get to the no-loss-or-gain calorie number. This baby step still has you monitoring calories every single day so that you don't go over your allowance.

You're still not eating out much, if at all, but you could be adding foods that have more calories or fat grams or sugar, etc from the supermarket as long as you know exactly how many calories you're eating and using your equation each day in order to maintain at your goal weight. Remember that it's not sugar, fat, or carbs that control your weight. It's CALORIES.

I suggest you keep using this baby step until you have a bunch more foods on your menu that you know you can eat with all of your other, healthier foods and still keep the calorie intake at the level it needs to be in order to maintain your weight. I think this step could take as short as 1 month and as long as 6 months. Remember, you're changing your entire life. It will still take a lot of time, and you have a lot of time to do it so stop complaining!

Baby step number 2 is where you could start adding fast foods back into your diet as long as you know exactly the calorie content in them and are still using your formula daily in order to maintain your weight.

Only today is this even possible. You can go to the fast-food restaurant official websites and pull their entire menus with the calorie amounts in every piece of food they push over their counters.

Now some of you are saying "wait a minute!" "Why are you letting us go back to fast foods if we're supposed to change our entire lifestyle and eat healthy for the rest of our lives?" Well I've got two answers to that question. First, like I said before, you don't necessarily see thin people eating only healthy foods do you? Second, you'll find out soon enough that, just because I'm letting you add fast food back in doesn't mean it'll be anything you want! In order to still maintain your calorie levels, there are very few of these foods that you'll even be able to eat anyway!

Some fast food places, like Taco Bell for instance, have special menu items that are lower in calories if you ask for them at the counter (theirs are "Fresco" items). Others are incorporating lower calorie items into their everyday menus and using substitute side-dish items so you can choose not to have those high calorie fries.

So if you're going to be really careful, and very diligent on monitoring the calorie levels per serving like you've grown so accustomed to doing, then go ahead and start adding some limited items in that group back into your diet. You'll find that you don't even like them as much as you used to, and that you might not even *want* to eat them very much anyway. But if you are one of those that still crave these things, then go ahead as long as you can monitor the *exact* calories.

I feel that you'll be on this step for at least several months before you'd want to move forward. This I call the step of experimentation. Keep experimenting with what you can and cannot add to your calories per day and maintain the calorie level needed to not gain weight. Continue to use Stage 4 methodology in order to lose any weight you may gain.

My research has shown me that it is supposed to take 3500 calories to gain 1 pound. This can be deceiving, because you may gain weight without going that far over your calorie levels. That's why this step can be frustrating. The added sodium in the things you've refrained from eating for so long is what's causing you to gain water weight and making you doubt your methods and results.

You'll learn after awhile that this water weight will come right back off in a few days using Stage 4, but that's why I am suggesting you do this experimentation for a long time over many months so you can get your mind used to the gain and loss of water weight based on those foods you're eating that aren't on the original accepted list.

Baby step number 3 is added in order for you to condition yourself to change the number of calories you eat at certain meals in order to allow for larger calories at a different meal or perhaps a dessert or after-dinner snack.

Here is where you're going to plan ahead for after breakfast (I NEVER recommend lowering your calories at breakfast no matter what you're planning for later in the day. You NEED those morning calories to fuel your metabolism!) those meals that may be larger, or where you can't count calories, and compensate by deducting foods from your menu at those meals.

For example, let's say you know you're going to have a large lunch due to a business function or due to a fellow employee's going away party, etc. You would plan your dinner to be a lot lower in calories to allow for the bigger lunch.

It's usually the other way around. You have dinner plans, or there's a family function after work, etc. You would drop your lunch to a very low calorie level to allow yourself to have many more calories at dinner and still meet the formula. Even if the foods you are going to eat at those functions cannot be analyzed for exact calories, you still will monitor the calories you've eaten (or are going to eat) for the rest of the day and take your best guess as to how many calories you're eating during the anomalous meal.

This will help you practice the fine art of moderation that you're getting used to. When you can't find out the exact calories of that meal, and you're so used to *knowing* how many calories you're eating, your mind should make you eat in moderation for fear of gaining weight that day or week.

If you find yourself pigging out like it's a cheat day or something, then your mind is not ready for the next baby step yet! Make sure you're not going crazy and eating too much when these situations occur. When you can get through these things regularly while keeping the eating in the proper moderation so that your weight doesn't go up (remember you're weighing yourself every day!) then you're ready to move forward.

I also do not recommend skipping lunch altogether, since eating 3 meals will keep your metabolism up throughout the day. However, if you MUST skip a meal for fear of going over your calorie level during a day such as above, go ahead and make it lunch. You don't want to skip dinner because it will be so hard for you to not eat late that night due to starvation!

Believe it or not, thin people do this almost subconsciously. They eat smaller meals throughout the day if they know they're going to have a big dinner, or have a bigger lunch if they know they can control what they're going to eat later. You've just never dealt with that before, so this step is necessary for you to add that to your mental arsenal in the fight for weight control.

These first 3 baby steps should take you a while to complete properly. Properly means that you're very comfortable with what you're doing and, most importantly, you can maintain your weight easily while doing that step.

You definitely should not move along if you can't say those things with certainty. If you've learned anything throughout this plan, you've learned that everything should be done gradually. You should take as much time as you can in order to assure that the principles you're using will stick with you permanently.

At this point you look great and feel great. You're going to stay that way for the rest of your life right? So what's a couple of months here and there going to mean in the long term? That's right…NOTHING. So stop worrying about how long it'll take. I performed these 3 baby steps for a total of about 6 months.

THE LAST OF THE BABY STEPS

Baby step number 4 is going to take the highest level of self-control you've ever exhibited, and you'll need to be at the mental state you'll need to keep for the rest of your life. The mental state must be that of a thin person. You must *believe* you are no longer an overeater, and that no amount of temptation is going to make you eat anywhere close to the way you used to back when you were overweight.

If this is the case, and you're truly ready, then the last step is to ***stop calorie counting***. YOU HEARD RIGHT! Stop counting. You know by now what you can eat at each meal and keep within your range. You're an expert at it! You even know through the previous baby steps how to add some fast foods and other luxury food items back into the plan while maintaining your proper weight and still eating very healthily.

You've learned how to adjust your day in order to plan for bigger meals or special events or plans. You've learned how to eat at those types of events ***in moderation*** so as not to throw off everything you've worked for.

In order to make this baby step work, you're still going to be monitoring something, just not calories. What you'll be monitoring is your weight, in pounds, on the scale at the same time every day. Now you're saying "I do that anyway!" That's right! Only now, you'll be using it as the gauge to judge whether you stuck with the program on the prior day or not.

Now for the first couple days, you'll gain a little water weight, and if you've been exercising, you've probably gained a little muscle weight as well. Remember, you're eating very well and taking calcium and a multivitamin, so you're burning fat every day, even if only a little. More of your weight is muscle now than it probably ever was before.

So I would wait for about 3 days before deciding you've gained too much and need to go back to Stage 4. After 3 days, you should be able to keep your weight on the scale each day at exactly what it was the day before simply by using your judgment and meal expertise to watch what you're eating during your 3 meals. You're not eating late, of course, and know your moderation techniques like the back of your hand.

Remember I said earlier that your goal now is to stay within plus or minus 5 pounds of your final goal weight. This is a great place to judge that on a daily basis. I would say once you've comfortably stopped counting calories, you could judge how you're doing on the maintenance plan by never going 8 pounds or more over your final goal weight. I give allowance for 3 to 5 pounds of water weight since you've added some more sodium-rich foods back into your diet.

8 pounds may sound like a lot, but for people who have been our size, that's nothing. For those of you that started at Stage 4 and wanted to lose just the vanity pounds, it may be a lot more, so you may want to keep that number within 3 pounds.

Is your mind comfortable with this? Are you truly ready to start living the rest of your life like a more normal person? Can you make it through 2 weeks straight while not counting calories and still staying at a consistent weight? If so, then congratulations! You're pretty much there! If not, then keep working at it!

You can always go back to the comfort zone of Stage 4 any time you need it in order to lose any excess weight back that you've gained. By now though, you shouldn't need to look at labels or count calories even on Stage 4. You should know exactly what you could eat for each meal to be at the exact calorie level you need to be to lose weight that week.

This is, in its basic form, the method you'll hopefully be using for the rest of your days in order to maintain your weight. I can't imagine having to use any other methods at all from now on.

Think about it. You're not counting calories anymore, eating mostly healthy foods for 3 meals each day, and when the foods aren't as healthy, you're eating them in moderation as if you had always been doing that.

You're weighing yourself every day. If you start to show a few more pounds, you lower your portions or only eat healthy foods up to your calorie level per day, which you now know almost instinctually. In case of emergencies, you can use Stage 4 to get back to your starting point, which only takes a few days to a week.

You're a thin person now!

CHEATING ON STAGE 5

So…up until now and throughout Stage 4, you truly looked forward to cheat days. Remember those days? Remember how you were still pigging out for a day or two and eating anything you wanted without consequence? Well those days are OVER.

Through the baby steps of Stage 5, you've weaned yourself off of those types of cheat days, and you've finally weaned yourself off of calorie counting as well.

Does this mean you can never cheat again? Of course not. It means that the *way* you cheat, even the whole *idea* behind cheating **MUST** have changed in order for you to be successful keeping your excess weight off for the rest of your life.

You've mastered the fine art of moderation during the last several months, and this is still the order of the day when it comes to cheating from now on. No longer can you allow yourself to cheat for a whole day or even a half-day. When you first start cheating again, even letting your mind *think* you're cheating, you need to micromanage it just as you did when you were losing the weight in the first place.

I'm not talking about counting calories again or anything like that. I just mean it has to go one step at a time. So the first time you cheat, it should be just *one* item of indulgence that day. I'm talking about *one* piece of cheesecake, *one* candy bar, *one* cheeseburger, or *one* ice cream creation at Cold Stone Creamery.

Now some of you are saying, "Wait a minute!" "This is exactly what I was during doing the baby steps!" "This is just an exercise in moderation!" **NO**. That's not what I'm getting at here. The difference is subtle, but it's there. During the baby steps, I was having you add other foods back into your diet in moderation **as part of your daily calorie intake**. I was also having you create allowances for events or plans in your day in order to compensate for higher-calorie meals that were mostly out of your control.

What makes this different is that, in your mind, there is no other reason for you to do what you're doing. There are no other plans, no unforeseen events, and no outside pressures on you to have the item in question pass by your lips.

That's why your mind should see it as *cheating*. You just simply decided you were going to have that item that day as an **indulgence.**

This should make sense to you. What your mind will see as cheating now is anything outside of a planned meal or part of your day. At first, if you keep it to one thing, you'll notice that it doesn't really hurt your weight at all (unless that one thing was HUGE, but you should have stopped doing that a long time ago!). This is why I suggest the one thing only rule until you're comfortable.

This doesn't mean one thing every single day! It means only once in a while. That's why it's called ***cheating***. If you did it every day, it would be a habit, and you'd gain the weight back.

Many of you will end your cheating here at this level. Hopefully, most of you won't even want to cheat anymore at any levels higher than the one-item rule. Your bodies and minds have turned a corner a long time ago now, and you are living the life of a thinner person like you always wanted to.

Isn't it great! This is where I'm at now. I don't even want to cheat like I used to. It makes me feel terrible the next day, and I have to go back to Stage 4 to lose the weight, and at this point, I don't like Stage 4 anymore!

Cheating at any level higher than the one item rule is up to you. If you do, I would suggest no more than one meal. I understand that there are holidays, vacations, family gatherings, cookouts, etc. However, you only need to watch the thin people you know at those types of things and you'll see how they do it.

They may eat at that one meal, and in moderation at that, and then they don't indulge in anything else the rest of the day.

This should be your guide. You should be able to watch other thin people and use them as your guide on how to eat at functions and on vacation. Talk to them. Try to get more of an understanding every day so you can keep converting your mind into that of a thin person even more than it already is.

You can always fall back on the fact that if you gain too much weight, you'll know exactly how to take it off using Stage 4 methodology. I've used it as a crutch many times, and I'm sure I'll continue to do so for the rest of my life. Because I know that this is foolproof, I am comfortable that I will never again be overweight, and you should be too.

FINAL WEIGHT-LOSS WORDS

What I really want to say here at this point, and I've already said it many times, is CONGRATULATIONS! I cannot stress enough how proud you should be of yourself for what you've done. I'm just very happy that I could show you the way and help you reach your dreams.

I know that if you've stuck with my plan and my advice as I've laid it out for you, that you are as thin as you want to be, while feeling better and healthier than you ever have before.

You may have even been checked out by your doctor during a physical or had blood work done for insurance or something like that and heard how much of a perfect specimen you are now. Isn't that something!

For me, I still can't get over how healthy my doctors say I am. I know I was probably a heart attack waiting to happen a few years ago, but now my cholesterol is low and I feel stronger and have more energy than I can every remember having. The added benefits to my sex life with my wife can also be seen as nothing but extremely positive!

I want to reiterate here that you should be proud that you did it the right way. I was sorry to have to tell everyone that there were no quick fixes when this plan began. If you've read a lot of the diet books out there, any worth their weight will tell you the same thing. It takes *time* to lose weight properly, keep it off, and change your lifestyle forever.

A lot of those books out there though will tell you that you absolutely must incorporate an exercise plan into your life in order to lose the weight and keep it off. I hope you've realized and are happy that this isn't necessary. Many of you have done what I did, and changed your life while only exercising very moderately, if at all, and certainly not on any standardized schedule.

For most of you, it's been at least a year, maybe 2 years, in getting to this point. That seems like a long time, but you now know you'll be able to do this forever. You now know that you are indeed a thin person. Enjoy all the benefits in life that being a thin person brings! They are numerous. People that have always been thin take them for granted. You will not.

When you see someone out there that was like you used to be and they're trying to change their lives, but don't know how, be sure to pass along your knowledge. You could even recommend this book to them if you're so inclined!

Most importantly, you can never forget where it is you've come from. Look at those old pictures from time to time. The people around you will have given up long ago on trying to break you of your new body. They changed from your biggest critics to your biggest fans.

Now, those people will start to forget everything that's happened, and you won't be getting that daily affirmation anymore about how thin you are and how great you look.

So I say again. You make sure you always keep in your mind how great you look and what you've accomplished. Don't worry…your reflection should keep reminding you!

Stage 6

Spicing Things Back Up

This is going to be a very short Stage! It's worth discussing though, no matter how briefly, how I've managed to keep my sanity and not eat the same things over and over again every single day in order to maintain my weight.

I'll admit that I don't really need the variety that I used to when I was heavy in order to keep myself happy, but let's face it, healthy foods can be boring. Simple chicken or fish dishes, the same old sandwiches for lunch, the same old yogurt and pudding cups for dessert, the same vegetable side dishes all the time, these things get monotonous.

In Stage 5, you started to add other things back into your diet, and you learned about moderation. The reason moderation was so important was that those things you were adding were not healthy foods! They were things you shouldn't be having, but weren't going to mess up your diet or your weight if you added them in moderation.

What I'm talking about now is not adding or subtracting things that you want to eat because they were previously off limits, but adding variety to the healthy foods you've been eating as your mainstay to healthy weight loss and maintenance.

There Can Be Variety In Healthy Eating

Believe it or not, this is true. Before I became a thin person and converted my mind to that of a thin person, I never would have believed it. If you start using resources and checking into it, you'll find that there are quite a lot of ways out there to change up the things you're eating in order to keep your taste buds happy and keep the variety of foods in your life alive.

I am not going to use this as an opportunity to put a bunch of recipes in this book. I don't like stealing other people's ideas or creations. In fact, I'm imploring you to seek those out on your own. I'm just telling you that they're out there.

Start looking at those magazines at the checkout counter in your supermarket. Many of them have amazing recipes that will show you how to create great tasting dishes out of the same healthy foods you were using to lose weight in the earlier Stages of my plan.

You may even start subscribing to some of those magazines in order to get fresh ideas and recipes more often. I use snippets of what I see from time to time in order to create new things to keep some new flavor in my diet. I try to only use recipes I see that include the items and spices that I already have in the house.

I don't like to have to make special shopping trips in order to get things for one specific recipe. However, If I like something very much, I'll get the items needed for that recipe, and will find that having those items in the house increases the number of recipes I can use from that point forward!

Another great thing about most of these publications and the recipes they contain these days is that they usually have the nutritional information per serving listed at the end of each recipe! Imagine…you could even incorporate these into Stage 4 if you wanted to! This is so different from how things used to be.

So you can pick and choose between recipes that not only sound good to your particular brand of taste, but would also fit into your specific calorie range per day!

I hope you get as excited about these things as I do. Since I'm a thin person now, these are the things I think about and look forward to as regards the food I eat.

You're A Cook Now...Right?!

What this Stage is alluding to is that you *can* cook, and you **needed** to cook in order to get through this entire plan. I know you may have only been using the stovetop, oven, indoor grill, and the microwave all this time, but I'm here to tell you that usually those are the only things you'll need anyway.

Most of the recipes you're going to find out there are easily prepared in the oven or on the stovetop and usually take only 10–30 minutes of your time to prepare anyway.

Many more methods of speeding up these recipes are being presented out there as a common theme for our busy lives these days is how to cook healthy meals in a very short period of time.

It seems that everything out there is created in our favor! All you needed to do was get used to the idea that you can cook for yourself instead of always having your food prepared at restaurants or in packages from the store.

By now, you're probably the cook in the family, preparing healthy meals every night for dinner not just for yourself, but for your whole family. Maybe you've even helped your spouse or children lose weight right along with you all this time.

If you've had someone else prepare your meals all this time, then you're very lucky. You need to make sure that person never leaves your side for the rest of your life. Treat that person like a Queen or King and make sure you tell them you love them every day. They are the ones who'll change up the recipes and keep you below the calorie levels.

It's very rare though. For the rest of us, just do it yourself! Be proud that you now are a good cook (or at least an edible one!) and that you can sustain yourself and your meals every day to keep yourself thin.

One easy way for those of you who aren't great cooks to keep up the variety in your diet is to go ahead and use those lean frozen dinners at your supermarket. I know I was negative about pre-packaged foods before. That was when you were overweight and were eating the bad ones!

I'm talking about checking out all of those creations made for people on a calorie budget. There are many different brands and many different food creations to choose from. Pick your favorites and mix things up a little at lunch or dinnertime.

I don't think it's as fun as cooking for yourself, and I also believe you get less food and higher sodium amounts using those frozen dinners. However, I can't whip up orange chicken or some of those great Chinese food dishes in my kitchen, so I can understand using them from time to time. It almost simulates eating restaurant food if you find a really good one.

Last but not least, if you have a time crunch due to the million things that go on in our daily lives, these dinners can come in handy.

So you see…you either cook a lot or you don't. In this day and age, it doesn't always really matter!

CHEATING ON STAGE 6

Are you still cheating? Just kidding! You're always going to want to indulge in something every once in a while. Only now, I shouldn't have to guide you anymore.

You know from Stage 5 how to do it. You weaned yourself off of cheat days and cheat half-days. You learned moderation and the one-item-per-day rule.

So the only thing I have to tell you here is to simply keep doing what you have been doing, and what works for you, for the rest of your days. Always remember where you came from, and that you now have the mind of a thin person, and you'll never go back to the way it was.

It doesn't hurt though that your mind still feels really guilty when you have that ice cream. It still does, right? I think that's your mind's way of giving you that reminder. I don't think you'll ever be able to get rid of that guilt. It'll keep you honest. Be happy when you feel it!

Those out there who have always been thin don't understand what that guilty feeling is all about. It's because they have always instinctually moderated their intake of bad foods. Maybe they were raised that way, I don't know.

Now you're more on par with them as to how you live your life, but you still have that mental guilt to keep you in check. Who knows…as you get older and so do they, you may stay thin and they may start to gain weight!

REMEMBER TO SPOT CHECK

As you go forward with this part of your life, you're definitely enjoying yourself! Isn't it amazing that you can eat the things you're eating, in the manner you're eating them, and be very happy every day doing it?

I know it is for me. I also know, as I pointed out near the end of Stage 5, that I must always remember where I came from, so I must incorporate a miniature plan that helps me make sure I never gain the weight back.

As I keep changing the recipes and meals in my daily diet in order to spice my meals up over and above the ordinary and plain stuff I ate a lot of when I was losing the weight, I've been continuing to weigh myself every day to be sure that my experiments aren't having a negative effect on all of my hard work.

Usually, that should be enough to be sure that you're going to maintain where you are. Sometimes though, I make extra sure by performing a spot check on the amount of calories I ate on a particular day.

Just simply wait until the end of the day, then go back and write up an exact calorie list of every item you ate that day, in the serving sizes you ate them, and their corresponding calorie amounts. Then total them up and see just where you were for that day. Plug the number into the formula and make sure it fell at or below your ideal caloric intake for a day based on your current weight.

For you who have followed my plan to the letter, this should be very easy! If you're incorporating foods now based upon an expanded menu that you created from foods and recipes that had nutritional information per serving calculated for you by magazine articles, you already have all of the information you'll need to do this.

For those of you still calculating each item from their own labels or from the internet website of your choice, it'll be even easier for you. If you become expert at judging things without calculating calories at all, then consider it a memory jogger of how to do all of that again in case you need it in the future.

No matter what the case, I recommend doing this spot check about once every 6 weeks in order to be sure you're staying with the program as you should. If you haven't been gaining any weight, you may think this isn't necessary, and you may be right. However, you might be right on the edge of starting a weight gain and not even know it.

If you're adding foods that are higher in calories without checking, one day you may end up changing your combinations of foods in such a way as to push you over the daily calorie level, and you'll start to gain weight. Now you'll catch it on the scale of course, but if you haven't been doing spot checks, you won't know *for sure* what caused the problem.

Therefore, you may have a struggle figuring out which of all of your new items to cut and which to keep, as well as which combinations of those foods you can have during a day. Spot-checking your foods every month and a half will keep you very safe from this happening.

Make sure you write down your spot checks and store them somewhere, so that if you have a weight gain and need to figure it out, you can look at the sheets and be able to calculate with surety which foods to cut back on or which combinations to avoid in order to keep your calories where they should be.

Again, many of you will find that you didn't really need to do this, and that's fine. It'll just give you that much more reassurance that you're an expert at your weight maintenance and give you that much more confidence going forward.

For the rest of you, you may not need it most of the time, but the first time you do need it, you'll be **extremely** thankful that I asked you to do it!

When it comes to keeping myself looking this great after all of that long and sometimes agonizing work, I don't mind having to do this little bit of extra paperwork. You shouldn't either.

Conclusion

I hope you've enjoyed the journey as much as I did presenting it to you. I lost a lot of weight and have kept it off for a long time now.

I'm never going back to the way it was, and I'm sure you won't either. It took a long time, and nobody ever said it would be easy, but hopefully you found my methods easier than anything else you've ever tried.

That's why I decided to write this book and present my ideas to the public for their scrutiny. It worked for me, and it was so much easier on my mind and body than any of the other diets I had tried earlier in my life.

I still can't believe how much easier it gets seemingly every day due to the number of manufacturers out there producing more and better low fat and fat-free foods that we can all take advantage of.

It only makes sense in this era to take advantage of this and build a plan around utilizing those items in order to wean yourself off of the multitudes of bad foods out there.

This society is changing, slowly but surely, into one where all of those unhealthy foods will become a thing of the past. It may not be completely changed in our lifetimes, but I can envision a future where everything out there for a consumer to eat will be healthy, even if it tastes unhealthy.

Since we're not going to see that day however, at least we can keep up on the advances as they happen and use them to our advantage to keep the variety in our lives while staying thin and healthy.

If you've truly followed my plan from start to finish, then this book should be old and dog-eared by now, having been used as a reference for at least a year, if not 2 years or more. Hopefully you've seen that it's all you needed, and that it covered all the bases.

I firmly believe that no doctor out there could read this and say it's not healthy. I know that I did it and am healthier than I have ever been. I realize that many would prefer a rigid exercise regimen in order to maintain a healthy weight and lifestyle, so I'm sorry to disappoint there.

I'm sure you're not sorry though. I thought it was about time a plan came out that could be followed without having to have everyone commit to taking time out of their busy lives every day (or 3 times per week or whatever) in order to commit to exercising. I feel that doing that makes you have to perform twice the commitment. You commit one part to the diet, and another to the exercise.

We all know that twice the commitment equals twice the chances for failure. Anyway, I didn't fail, and neither did you. Please, whatever you do, don't go back to the way you were before. It means a lot to your health and longevity, and it makes it a lot easier to put on a bathing suit also!

Enjoy your new life. Look at your reflection and smile. When you get those extra glances from the opposite sex, tell yourself you're never going to change! Thank you for coming along for the ride!

Before And After Photos

I won't have to tell you which are which!

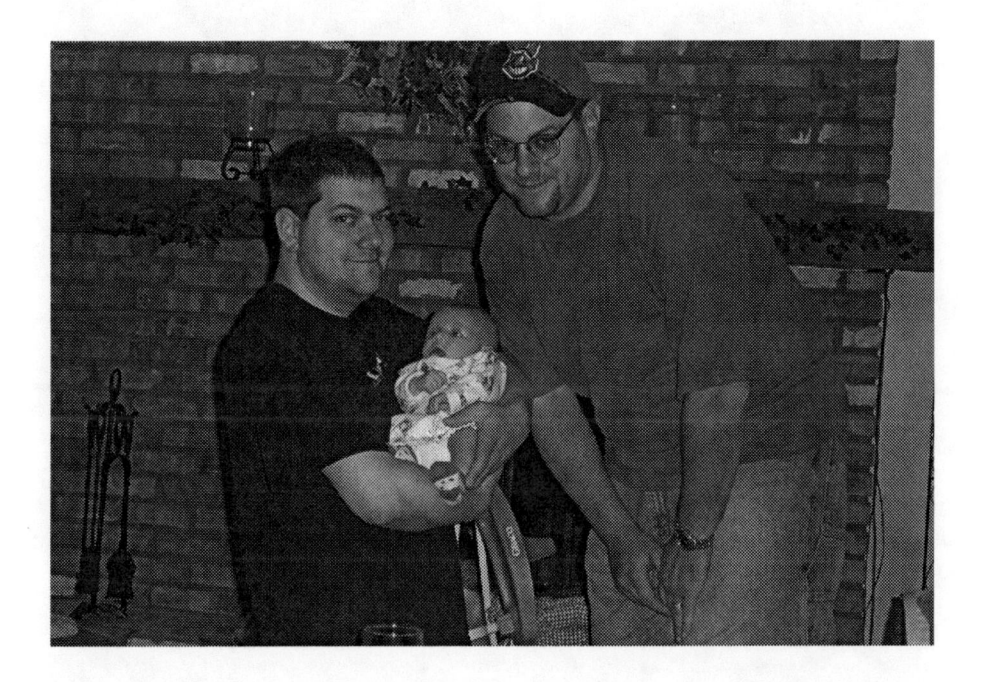

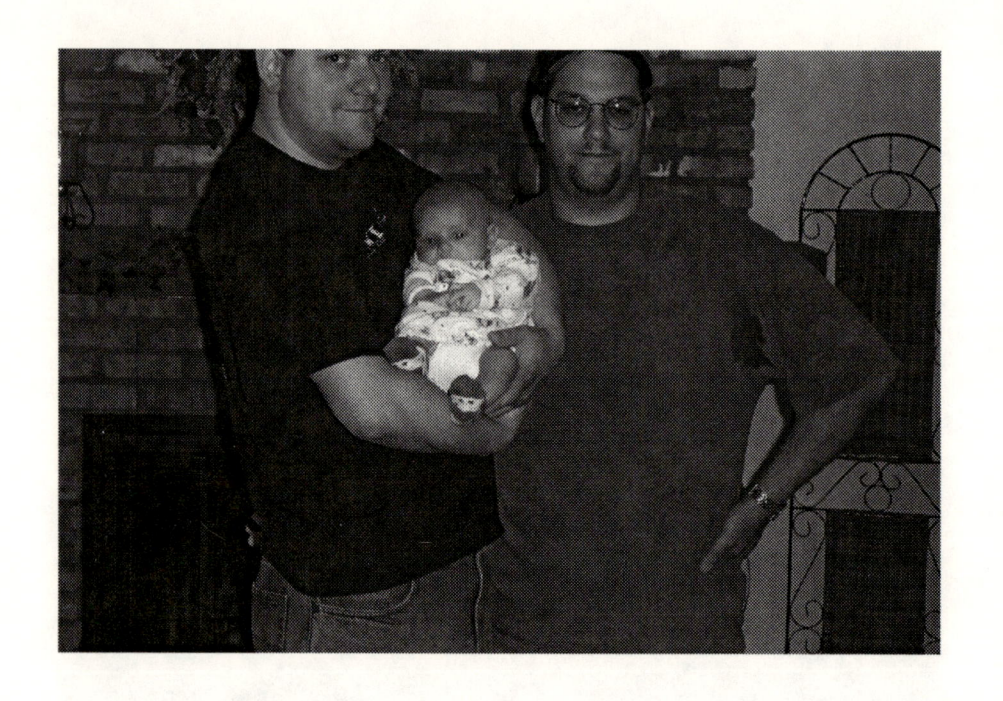

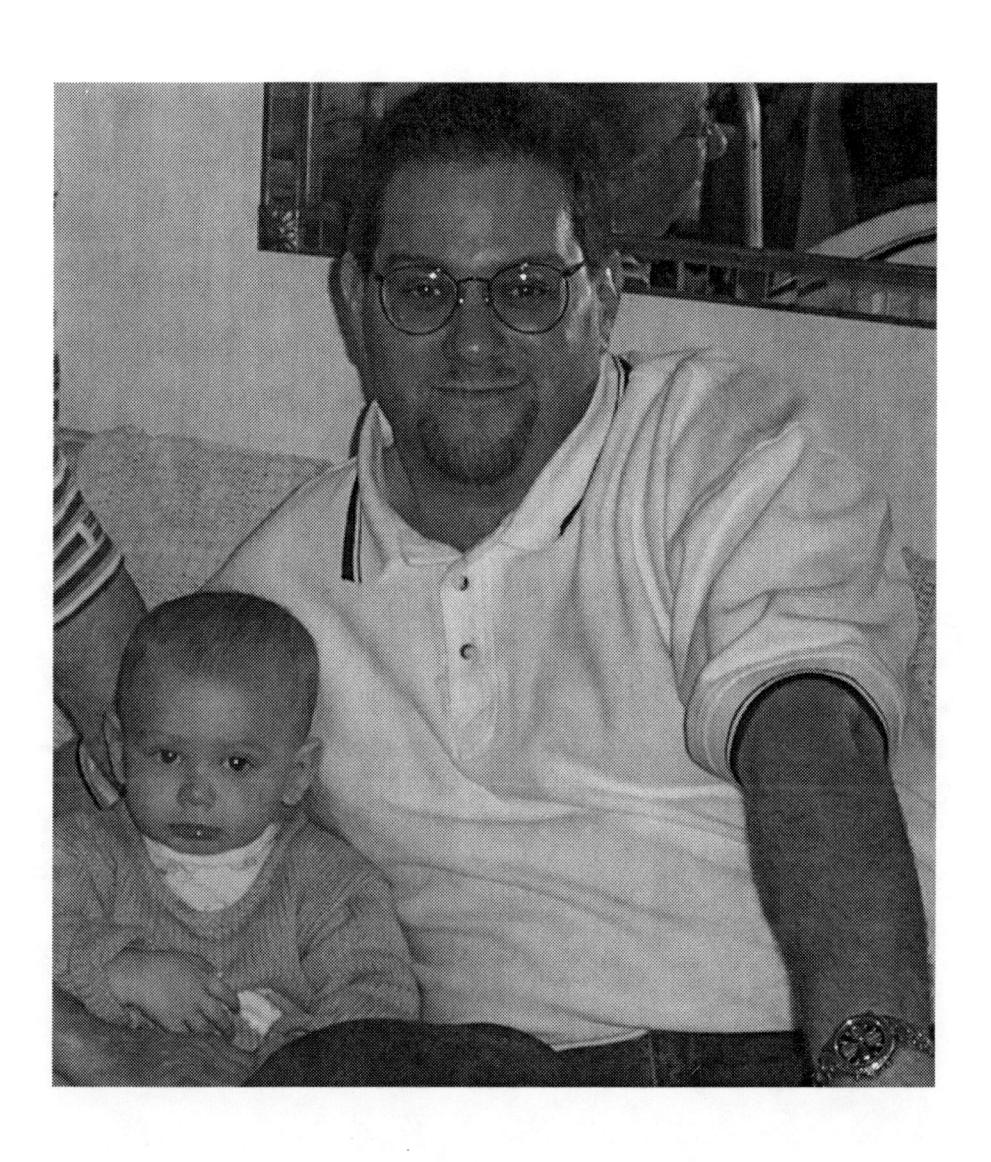

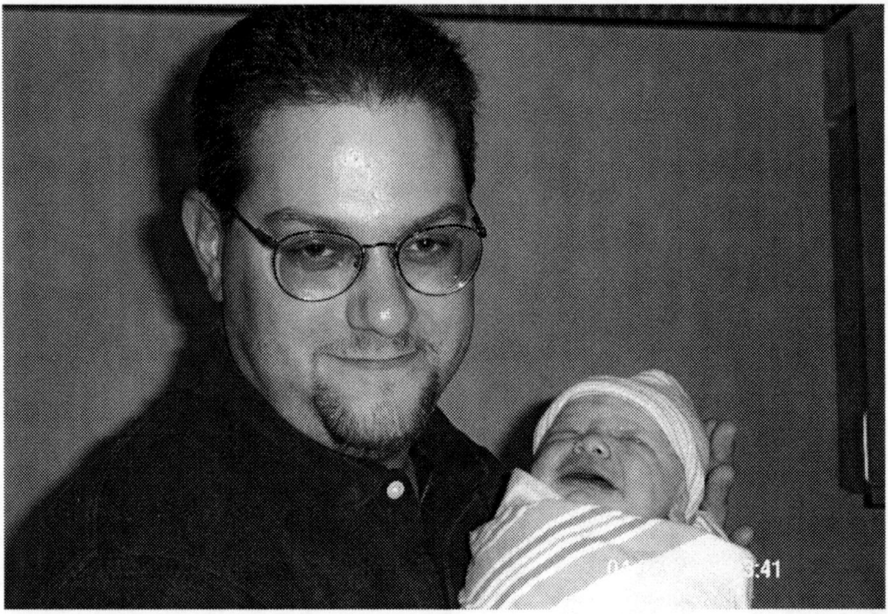

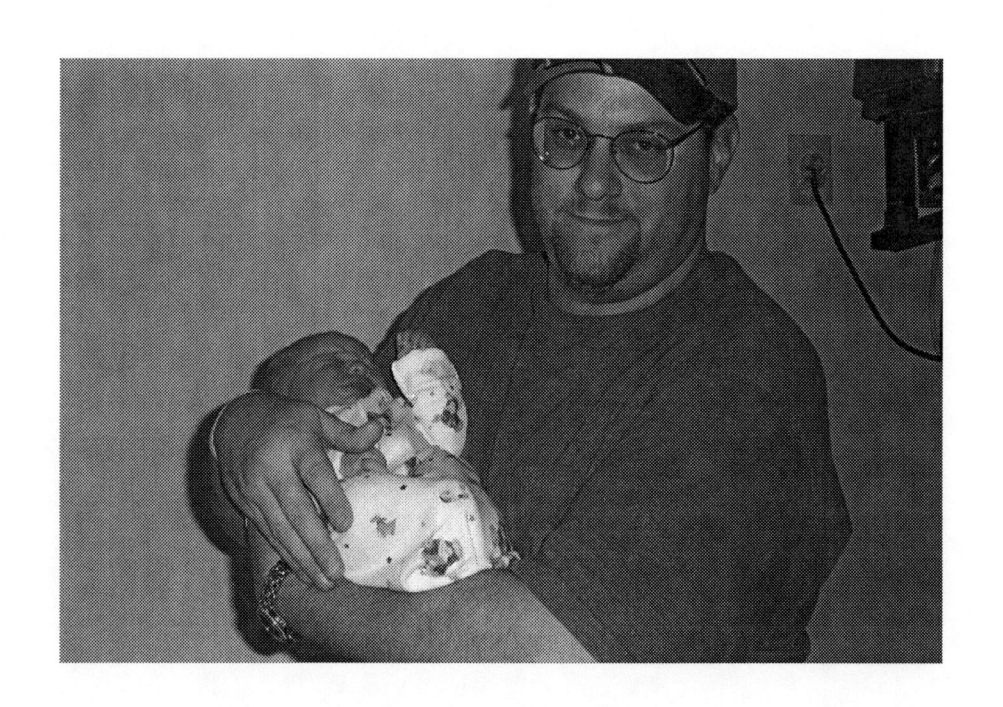

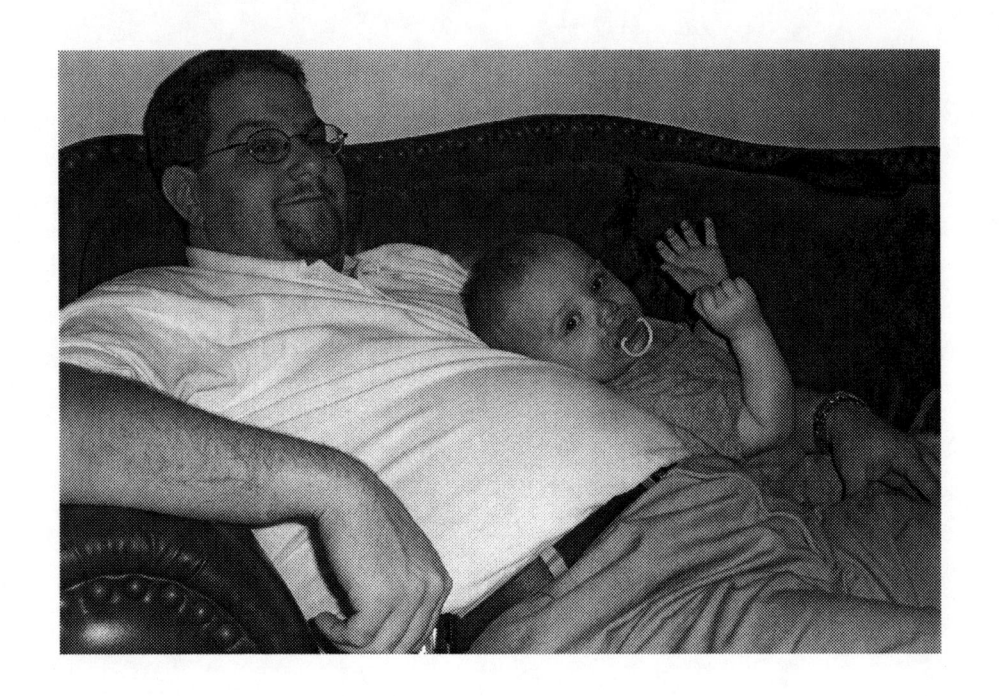

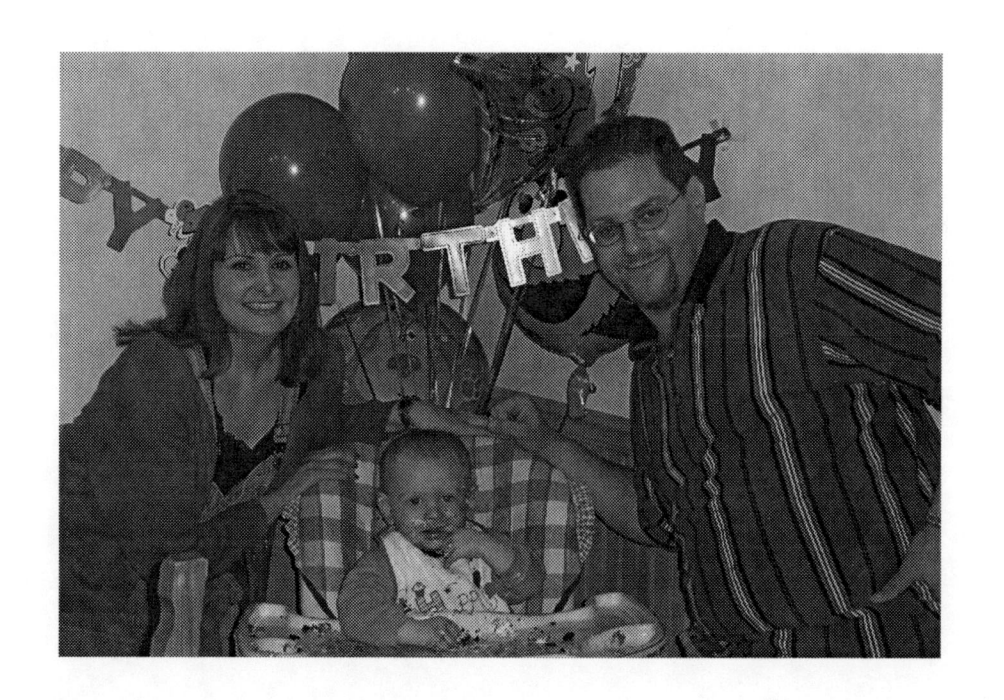

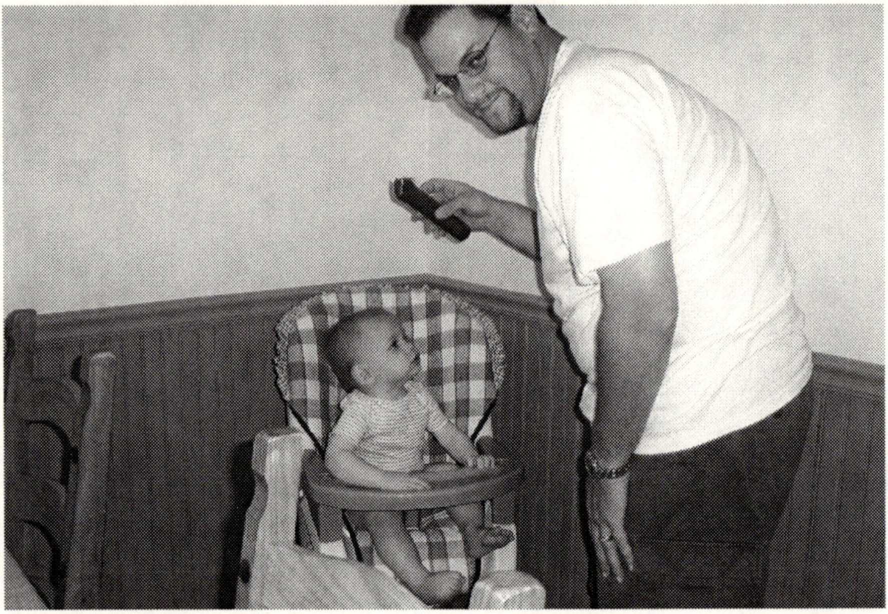

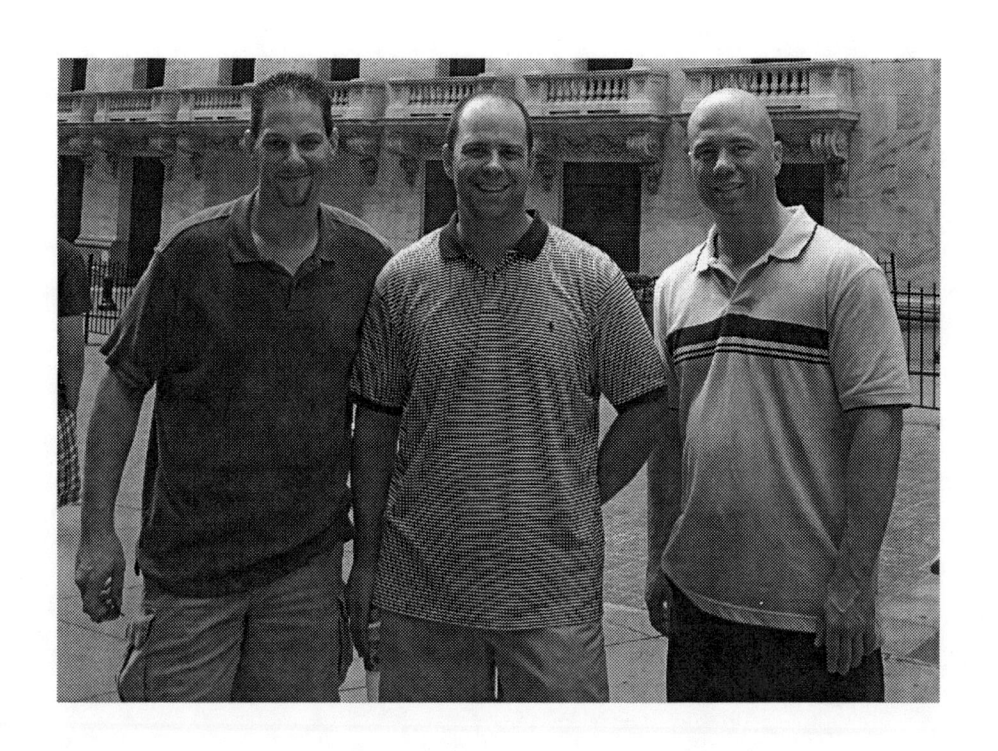

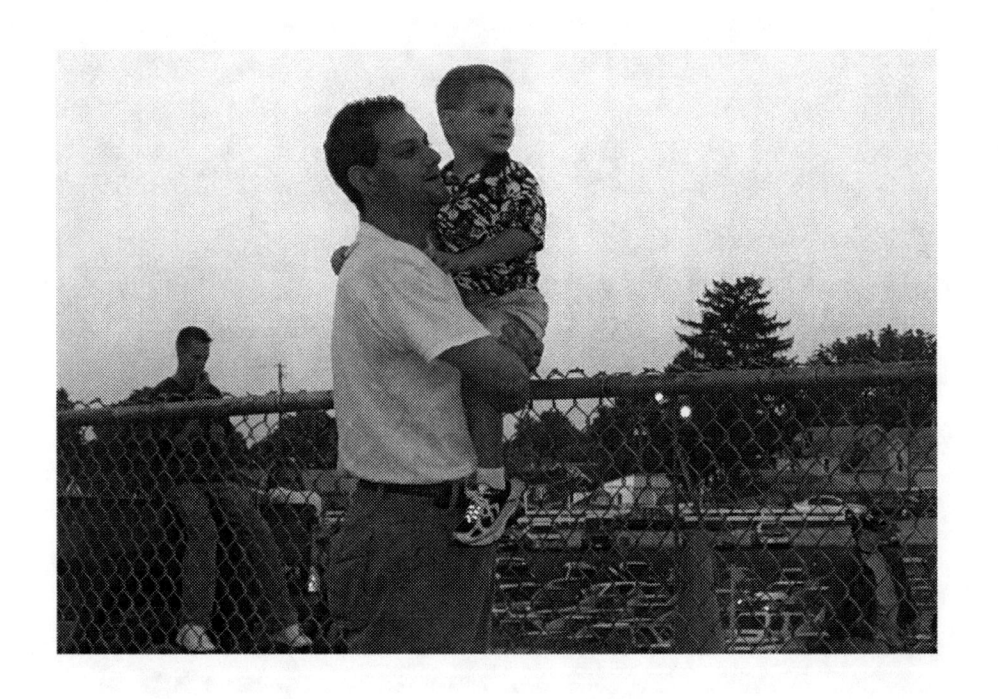

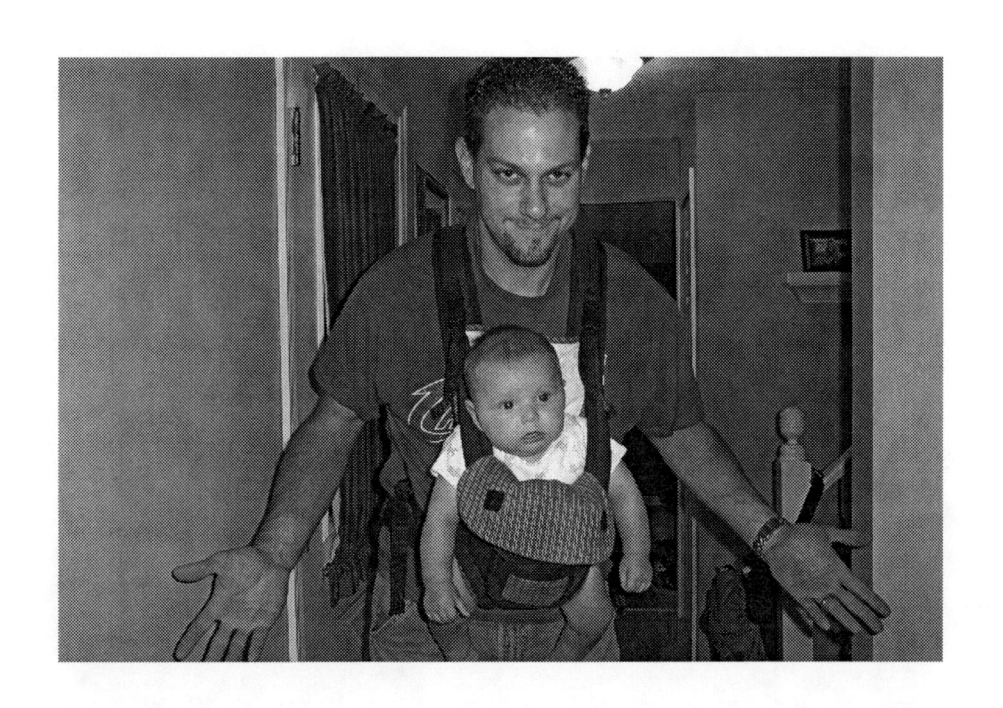

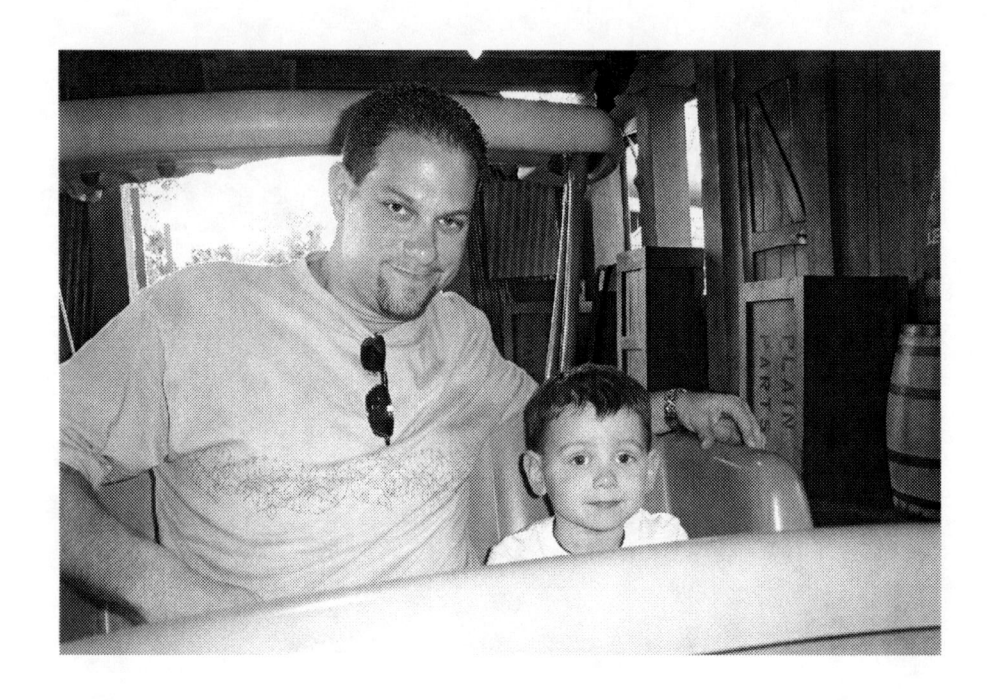

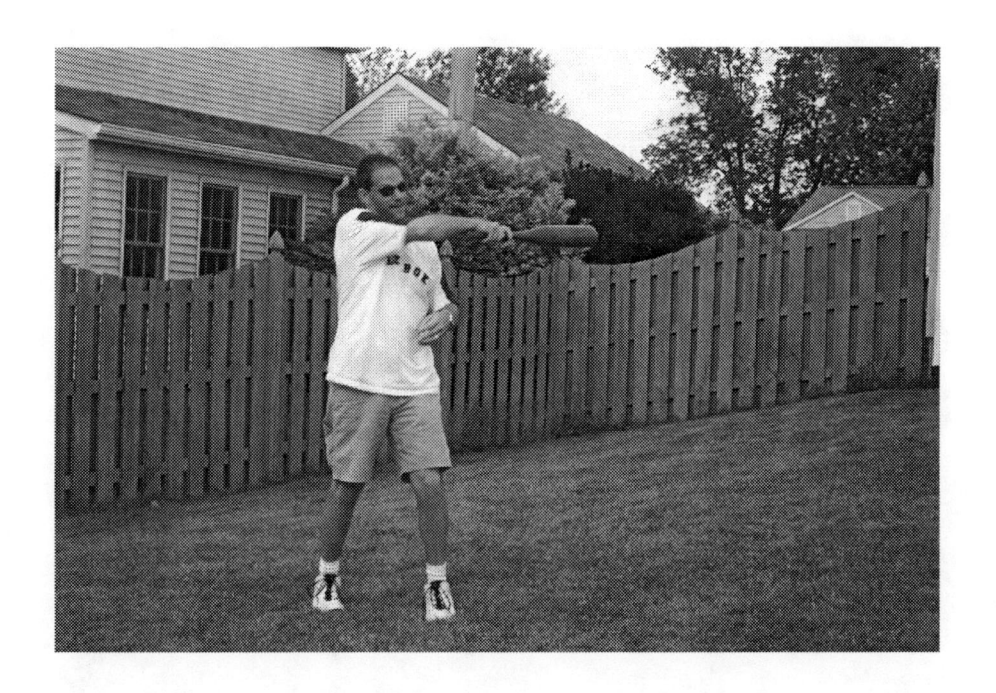

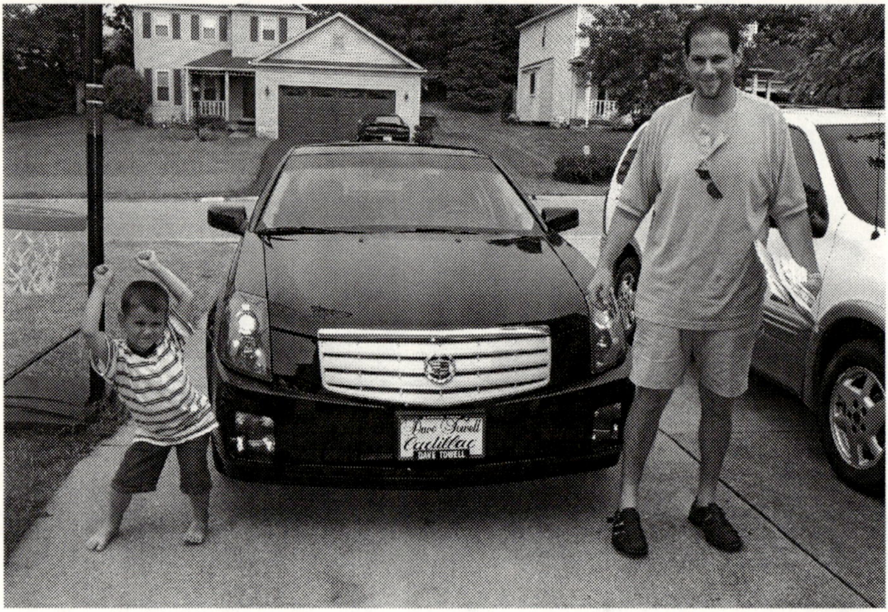
Dave Towell
Cadillac
DAVE TOWELL

978-0-595-41884-8
0-595-41884-8